Breast Cancer

Terry   is Consultant Oncologist and Honorary Senior Clinical
Lecture.   'versity of Birmingham. He is also Medical Editor for the
cha.. y M.   Cancer Support. He is a former Dean of the Faculty of
Clinical On.   / at the Royal College of Radiologists, and has written
more than a hundred papers for the medical press. He is also the author
of *Coping with Breast Cancer* (2006), *Coping with Radiotherapy* (2007),
Reducing Your Risk of Cancer (2008), *The Cancer Survivor's Handbook* (2009)
and *Coping with Chemotherapy* (second edition, 2011) all published by
Sheldon Press.

Overcoming Common Problems Series

Selected titles

A full list of titles is available from Sheldon Press,
36 Causton Street, London SW1P 4ST and on our website at
www.sheldonpress.co.uk

Overcoming Common Problems Series

Overcoming Common Problems Series

Overcoming Common Problems

Breast Cancer
Your treatment choices

DR TERRY PRIESTMAN

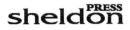

First published in Great Britain in 2013

Sheldon Press
36 Causton Street
London SW1P 4ST
www.sheldonpress.co.uk

British Library Cataloguing-in-Publication Data
A catalogue record for this book is available from the British Library

ISBN 978-1-84709-268-7
eBook ISBN 978-1-84709-269-4

Typeset by Fakenham Prepress Solutions, Fakenham, Norfolk NR21 8NN
First printed in Great Britain by Ashford Colour Press
Subsequently digitally printed in Great Britain

eBook by Fakenham Prepress Solutions, Fakenham, Norfolk NR21 8NN

Produced on paper from sustainable forests

Contents

Introduction

Let's begin with some good news: in the United Kingdom today more than 8 out of every 10 women who are told they have breast cancer will be cured. Finding out that you have breast cancer is a devastating shock and triggers an avalanche of fears and concerns. But with modern-day treatment the odds are in your favour and the chances are that you will be all right. Although there may be many ups and downs along the way, eventually life will get back to something like normal.

There are many different ways to think about life when you have been told you have breast cancer. One way of looking at it is to see it as a journey. At its most personal level that journey is one of self-discovery: how will you cope with knowing you have a life-threatening illness? What reserves of strength or unsuspected weaknesses will surface as you work your way through treatment? Will your feelings about those you love and care for change because your life has been thrown off course? Will your priorities, your ambitions, your beliefs or your faith change? These are just some of the deeply emotional issues that having cancer will lead you into, and everyone will respond in their own way.

But alongside this complex journey of ever shifting inner feelings is another more obvious but equally challenging path – the journey through your treatment; a road you will travel passing many ups and downs until finally, we hope, you are cured. In early breast cancer there are many different routes for that treatment journey running along different courses from the starting point of diagnosis to the finishing line of being cured and knowing your cancer won't come back.

Along those routes there are a number of major crossroads; places where decisions have to be taken as to which way to go – which treatments to choose from a number of possibilities. In the past, most women would not have realized when these important points were reached because they were simply told by their doctors what should happen next. The decision about their direction of travel had been made for them without their even knowing there was the chance of a choice. They were led blindfold past the crossroads, not realizing they could have gone in another direction.

Times have changed. Now the emphasis is on shared decision-making. Doctors are increasingly encouraged to involve their patients in choices about their treatment, and this is especially so in breast cancer. The focus is on giving you enough information to be able to make choices about what happens to you. At least that is the theory – the ideal. Sometimes it works but sometimes it doesn't. Some doctors feel they should protect their patients from the difficulty of making major decisions about their treatment and simply tell them what to do, or at least steer them firmly in a particular direction. Some people feel they cannot cope with making choices, or want to trust their doctor's experience and knowledge and so ask them to make the decisions without telling them what their options are.

If you do want to be involved in making decisions about your treatment and if you are offered options by your doctor then in order to make the right choice you need information. These days this is widely available. First of all your medical team, your expert nurses and doctors, will tell you about the different treatments and their side effects. They will usually back this up with written information – booklets and factsheets from excellent organizations like Macmillan Cancer Support, Breast Cancer Care or Cancer Research UK. And of course there is always the Internet. There is also now a new scheme from the Department of Health, which has introduced 'information prescriptions' that give every person with cancer selected items of information from currently available publications, tailored to meet their own needs. However, like the information from the different cancer charities, your information prescription will only give you facts and figures; it won't tell you what you need to do. That is still up to you.

This sounds like an ideal system – a policy from the Department of Health that seeks to encourage women with breast cancer to have a say in their treatment and puts systems in place to give them the facts they need to make their choices. But does it work? In many places, for many women, the answer is probably yes. But for some years now I have held regular workshops for the charity Breast Cancer Care, talking to women who have, or have had, breast cancer and giving them the chance to ask questions about their illness and treatment. What has surprised me is how many of those women either have not been given the facts about their treatment and the choices they have, or have had, things explained to them in ways they have found confusing and unhelpful. What is more, many women have never had a clear explanation of why a particular type of treatment might be needed, what it is intended to do and what might happen if they decide not to have it.

The last point is a tricky one: saying no to any type of treatment if you have breast cancer is a brave and maybe foolhardy thing to do. It is a potentially life-threatening condition and if a treatment is offered, to refuse it could have disastrous consequences. But breast cancer is a very complicated illness and the range of treatments you might have is huge. For many women a number of these treatments are absolutely vital if a cure is to be possible; they are quite literally life-saving. But for other women some treatments are less important – they are, if you like, the icing on the cake, optional extras; their benefits are far less certain and they may make little or no difference to the chance of stopping the cancer coming back. This would not matter if those treatments were problem-free, but often they can have side effects, and these can vary from being mildly irritating to highly distressing or even life-threatening. In this situation there is a balance to be struck between the positive value of that treatment in increasing your chance of cure and its negative impact on your quality of life.

I am sure that any breast cancer specialist reading the last paragraph would say that they always discuss the pros and cons of treatment with the women they look after at all times throughout their treatment, and explain why a particular therapy is, or is not, a good idea and how important, or unimportant, it is to carry on with a treatment even if it is causing troublesome side effects. If you have a doctor like this then you probably don't need this book. But I'm afraid my experience of talking to hundreds of women with breast cancer is that they either don't get this input from their medical team or get in such a way that they can't understand it and are too confused, or even too frightened, to make choices about their care.

What I hope to do in the chapters that follow is explain where you will arrive at those vital crossroads on your breast cancer journey when decisions have to be made about treatment. I will also say something about the different types of treatment that might be on offer at each of these points along the way and talk about why those treatments might, or might not, be necessary and their benefits and drawbacks.

There are no absolute rules about right and wrong treatments in breast cancer. Various organizations produce official guidelines for breast cancer specialists, suggesting what might be the best treatment options in different situations at different points in time, but what these guidelines cannot and do not take into account is *you*. Each of us is an individual and each of us has our own view on life, what it means to us, and how we want to live it. Who we are, who we care about and what we care about will affect how we feel about different treatment choices. For instance, one woman may feel that being as certain as possible of getting a cure is the only thing she cares about – no matter what the treatment involves, whatever the side effects, whatever the inconvenience and stress, however long it goes on for; all that is a small price to pay. But another woman may put her quality of life centre stage and be more selective – picking and choosing only those treatments that she feels offer the greatest chance of a benefit and saying no thank you to others that have less likelihood of making a difference to her chance of cure.

The treatments used to cure breast cancer are surgery, radiotherapy, chemotherapy, hormone therapy and newer targeted drugs. With each of these the first choice is between having or not having the treatment. If you say yes then other choices have to be made: which sort of operation to have, which drugs to take? In the stressful atmosphere of an outpatient clinic, thinking straight about your options and making decisions can be nigh-on impossible and you should always be given thinking time – the opportunity to go over things in your own mind and talk them through with friends and family. This may lead you to your decision or it may lead you to questions you want to ask in order to get everything properly clear. I hope this book will help you through this process. It won't tell you what to do but it may fill in some of the gaps in the information you have been given, it might answer some of your questions and it may even give you some reassurance and more confidence as you travel your cancer journey.

Before we can look at your options and decisions in the treatment of your breast cancer we need to cover some basic facts about breast cancer, and that's what we'll do in the next chapter.

1

Key facts about breast cancer

When you are first diagnosed with breast cancer it is almost always in a breast clinic at the hospital, where all the staff there, the doctors and nurses, will be specialists in breast cancer. This is obviously a good thing because it is important for you to get expert care and attention. But it does mean that although the people on the clinical team have years of experience of dealing with breast cancer, they will sometimes forget that you don't know a lot about what breast cancer actually is and how it behaves, and they will often use words or talk about ideas that you simply don't understand. This can leave you confused and uncertain, which is a bad thing for at least two reasons: first, it adds to the fear and concern you will almost certainly have when you are first told you have cancer; and second, if, as is increasingly common these days, you are invited to make choices about your treatment this can be very difficult if you don't really understand the basic facts to help guide you through those choices. This chapter describes some of the key facts about cancer in general – and breast cancer in particular – in the hope that it will shed light on some of the things that doctors and nurses might have said that were puzzling or just plain incomprehensible.

What is cancer?

Our bodies are made up of billions of cells. Throughout life these cells will wear out and die. So every day we make millions of new cells to replace the old cells that are lost. This process is very finely controlled so that exactly the right number of new cells is made to balance the old cells that have gone. But sometimes things go wrong and too many new cells are made. If this continues then, over time, a swelling or growth will develop in a particular part of the body. These growths are called tumours. Tumours may be either benign or malignant. If the tumour is malignant then it is a cancer.

Most cancers begin as a single growth in a particular part of the body. This is called the primary cancer. The primary cancer is also described by the part of the body where it is located; so a cancer that begins in the breast is a primary breast cancer and a cancer that begins in the lung is a primary lung cancer. Cancers can occur in almost any part of the body and there are more than 200 different types.

There are two important differences between a benign tumour and a cancer. First, as a cancer grows it eats into and destroys the surrounding tissue. Doctors often talk about this as 'invasion', so a cancer is an invasive tumour. Benign tumours may grow to a large size but they do not invade the surrounding tissues and organs; they may push them out of the way or squeeze them but they do not eat into them. This means that if someone has an operation to take away a benign tumour then it can usually be removed quite easily. But if it is a cancer it will be much more difficult to see where the growth ends and normal tissue starts, so in order to take it away completely the surgeon will have to remove a margin of normal tissue around the cancer.

The second difference between a benign tumour and a cancer is that cancers can spread to other parts of the body but benign tumours cannot. This means that tiny clumps of cells can break away from a primary cancer and be carried by the lymph vessels or the bloodstream to nearby lymph glands or to organs like the liver, lungs, brain or bones. When a cancer spreads elsewhere these new cancers are called secondary cancers (secondaries or metastases). So if a primary breast cancer spreads to the lungs then the tumours in the lungs will be secondary breast cancers, or breast cancer metastases.

If a breast cancer spreads to the lungs then the secondary cancers will be made up of breast cancer cells and will behave like breast cancer, not like lung cancer. This can be quite confusing. For example, the media will often report that a particular celebrity has lung cancer when what he or she actually has is a secondary cancer – metastatic cancer that has spread to the lungs from a primary growth in another part of the body. Making this distinction is important because the behaviour, treatment and outlook for primary and secondary cancers are very different.

The lymph system

The lymph vessels are tiny thread-like tubes that drain colourless fluid called lymph from all the organs and tissues in the body. These vessels carry the lymph from a particular organ or tissue into nearby lymph nodes (which are also known as lymph glands). These are tiny bean-shaped structures that are normally quite small and difficult to see but that may become very enlarged and swollen if there is an infection or if a nearby cancer spreads into them.

The network of lymph vessels and lymph nodes runs throughout the body. Most of the lymph from the breast drains to lymph nodes in the armpit. The medical name for the armpit is the axilla, so doctors call these the axillary lymph nodes (Figure 1). The first of these lymph nodes that the lymph vessels reach after leaving the breast is called the sentinel node. When a breast cancer spreads through the lymph system, the sentinel node is almost always the first lymph node to be affected.

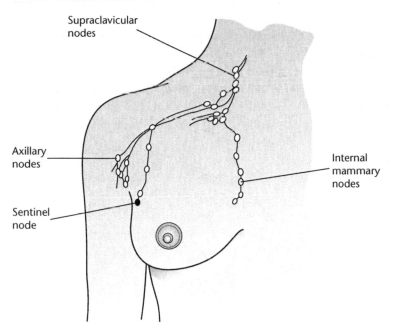

Figure 1 The position of different groups of lymph nodes (lymph glands) around the breast

Some of the lymph from the inner part of the breast (the part that lies closest to the breast bone) drains to lymph nodes that lie deep in the tissues alongside the breast bone. These are called the internal mammary nodes. Occasionally, cancer of the inner half of the breast will spread to these nodes but this is much less frequent than spread to the axillary lymph nodes.

The actual number of axillary lymph nodes varies from person to person but is usually somewhere between 20 and 30. Once a breast cancer has spread to these glands it may go on to spread to the next group of nodes, which lie just above the collar bone (the clavicle) on that side. These are called the supraclavicular lymph nodes. Spread of a breast cancer to these glands is relatively uncommon and usually only happens if there has been extensive involvement of the nearby axillary lymph nodes.

How does a breast cancer grow?

There is a vast amount of information, and even more disinformation, about what causes breast cancer, but we are going to bypass all that and jump to the stage when the breast cancer has first begun to develop.

The breast is made up of lots of tiny glands, the medical name for which is lobules (Figure 2). After a pregnancy these glands make breast milk, which is carried from the glands to the nipple through fine tubes called ducts. We now believe that most, if not

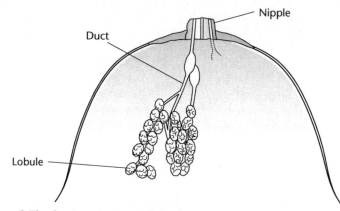

Figure 2 The basic structure of the breast

all, breast cancers begin in the cells lining the junction between the lobules and the ducts. Cancers that begin in cells lining a particular organ of the body are called carcinomas, so nearly all breast cancers are carcinomas because nearly all breast cancers begin in the lining cells where the lobules meet the ducts. Most of these cancers will begin to grow along the lining of the duct and so they are known as ductal carcinomas. Much less commonly the cancer will grow the other way, into the lobule, and this is called a lobular carcinoma.

At first, only the lining cells of the ducts or lobules are affected: the cancer has not begun to spread into the surrounding fatty and fibrous tissue of the breast; it has not begun to invade the breast and become an invasive cancer. This is what doctors call 'in situ' cancer. So a breast cancer that is within the cells that line the inner wall of the ducts but which has not begun to invade the surrounding breast tissue is a ductal carcinoma in situ, and the medical shorthand for this is DCIS. If the cancer has grown in the other direction and is involving the lining cells of the glands then it is a lobular carcinoma in situ or LCIS.

Usually, but not always, DCIS will eventually start to grow into the breast tissue around the duct; it will become an invasive breast cancer rather than an in situ breast cancer. This does not happen overnight. Although there is still a lot of uncertainty, experts suggest that DCIS may often be present for anywhere from 5 to 15 years before it turns into an invasive breast cancer.

Once the cancer has become invasive and begun to grow within the breast it will steadily increase in size. The speed at which breast cancers grow varies from person to person. As a general rule, breast cancers in younger women grow faster than those in older women, but this is not always the case. People tend to think of cancers as growing very rapidly, but even the fastest-growing breast cancers take about 3–4 months to grow from a lump measuring 2 cm from side to side to one measuring 3 cm from side to side, and with some slow-growing breast cancers this could take years. On average, the time taken for a breast cancer to grow from 2 cm across to 3 cm across is about a year.

The invasive breast cancer is the primary breast cancer. If it is not treated then at some time tiny clumps of cells will break off from this primary cancer and travel through the lymph vessels or the bloodstream to form metastases: secondary breast cancers. Usually the first place the breast cancer cells go to is the lymph nodes under the arm next to the breast (the axillary lymph nodes). When breast cancer cells travel through the bloodstream they most often form metastases in one or more of the bones, but the liver, lungs and brain are other parts of the body that are commonly affected. Different breast cancers can behave very differently. Some breast cancers will spread to the lymph nodes or other parts of the body when they are still very small. Others will reach a large size and still may not have formed any metastases.

Breast cancer in men

Men do get breast cancer and most of the information in this book is true for male breast cancer. There are some differences between breast cancer in men and women, and the most important of these are listed here.

- Breast cancer is more than 150 times more common in women than men: each year about 300 men in the UK are diagnosed with breast cancer whereas more than 45,000 women develop the disease.
- Breast cancer in men occurs at a slightly older age than in women: the average age at which women develop breast cancer is around 65 years but in men the average age is about 70 years.
- When it is first diagnosed, breast cancer in men is often at a more advanced stage, with about 4 out of 10 being stage 3 or 4 (see 'The stage of a breast cancer' in this chapter).
- When matched stage-for-stage the chance of cure is the same for men and women.
- Surgery for breast cancer in men almost always means a mastectomy.
- Rather surprisingly, male breast cancers are more often positive for oestrogen receptors (ER+) than breast cancers in women. Nine out of ten male breast cancers are ER+ and drugs like tamoxifen and aromatase inhibitors are very effective treatments.

To begin with these secondary cancers will be made up of only a small number of cells and will be microscopic – completely invisible and undetectable – and won't cause any symptoms or problems. Like the primary cancers, the growth rate of metastases from breast cancer is very variable: some may become large enough to be noticeable within 6 months to 1 year whereas others may not show themselves for several years.

The stage of a breast cancer

Staging a breast cancer is very important when it comes to deciding what treatment to recommend. The key parts of staging are working out the size of the primary breast cancer and whether it has spread to the lymph nodes or other parts of the body. Once a surgeon has removed your primary breast cancer the pathologist will measure the size of the growth and also look for signs of any spread to the lymph nodes. Other tests, such as scans or X-rays, may then be done to see if the cancer has gone anywhere else in the body. Once the medical team has all this information they can stage your cancer.

There are a number of different ways of recording the stage of a breast cancer and the most widely used of these is the 'TNM' system, which gives detailed information about the size of the primary tumour (T), the number of lymph nodes with signs of cancer (N) and whether there has been spread to other organs (M). This is a very complicated system but Table 1 gives an idea of how a very simple staging system could work.

Table 1 Cancer staging

Stage	Definition
1is	There is only DCIS or LCIS (*in situ* cancer)
1	There is an invasive cancer that has not formed any secondary cancers
2	The cancer has spread to one or more lymph nodes in the armpit
3	The cancer has invaded the skin of the breast or the muscle underlying the breast
4	The cancer has spread to other parts of the body

Early and late breast cancer

Another way to describe the stage of a breast cancer is to use words like 'early' and 'late'. Although these words are very often used by health professionals and the media, there is no universally agreed definition of the exact stages of breast cancer they cover, so they can mean slightly different things to different people.

Most health professionals would say that early breast cancer includes DCIS (and the much less common LCIS) and those breast cancers where the primary cancer is less than 5 cm across. If the cancer has spread to the lymph nodes under the arm it is still early but if it has spread anywhere else (to other lymph nodes or other parts of the body) then it is no longer an early breast cancer.

Late breast cancer, also known as advanced breast cancer, is the term usually used when there is spread to other parts of the body like the bones, liver, lungs or brain. Some health professionals also talk about this as metastatic or secondary breast cancer, so they will say, for example, that someone has secondary breast cancer in the bones, or metastatic breast cancer in the liver.

A third stage can also be used: locally advanced, or loco-regional, breast cancer. This includes those primary breast cancers that are larger than 5 cm across, primary breast cancers that have begun to invade either the skin overlying the breast or the muscle underneath the breast (on the wall of the chest), or those breast cancers that have spread to the lymph nodes above the collar bone (the supraclavicular nodes) as well as the lymph nodes under the arm.

A note on numbers

Much of the information that doctors rely on to help them give advice and make decisions about treatment for breast cancer is given in percentages. A clinical trial might show that 80 per cent of women were cured with a particular treatment, or another study might show that 25 per cent of women had sickness as a side effect when they were given a particular drug. These percentages simply mean that in the clinical trial 80 out of every 100 women treated were cured, and in the study 25 out of every 100 women who had the drug were sick. The percentages tell doctors the chances that a particular treatment will work or will cause side effects; in betting terms, they give doctors the odds.

This means that doctors tend to think in terms of percentages. But you are not a percentage, you are you. If we look at our example of the clinical trial, you can't be 80 per cent cured – either your treatment will lead to a cure or it won't. Either you will be one of the 80 out of 100 women who are cured or one of the 20 out of 100 who are not. The percentages spell out the chances of something happening or not happening, and those percentages can help you make up your mind about having or not having a particular treatment. But they don't say what will actually happen to *you*. You may be one of the lucky 80 out of 100 who are cured or one of the unlucky 20 out of 100 who are not.

Another thing to mention about percentages is how they are used to show the benefits of different treatments. Suppose you are told that with the treatment you are already having there is a 90 per cent chance of a cure but if drug X is added then your chance of cure goes up to 91 per cent. At first sight you may think anything that increases your chance of a cure is a good thing and you should have the drug. This may or may not be the case, but what those percentages really mean is that with the treatment you are already having, 90 out of every 100 women will be cured and having drug X only increases that number to 91 out of 100. This actually means that only 1 woman in every 90 will have any benefit from the extra treatment. In other words there is only a 90 to 1 chance that drug X will be of any help to you.

Let's look again at our example of a 25 per cent chance of having sickness as a side effect with a particular drug. People are often surprised when they have a side effect that they have been told there is only a 25 per cent chance of having. The fact that there is only a 1 in 4 chance of getting that side effect doesn't mean it can't happen; it means it is relatively unlikely but it still means there is a small chance that you will be unlucky enough to have that problem. Confusion can also arise over how often a side effect happens and how bad that side effect is – how upsetting it may be. The fact that a side effect only affects a small percentage of people, that only a few in every hundred get that side effect, doesn't tell you anything about how mild or how severe that side effect might be.

To keep things simple, in this book we will only use 'early' and 'late' breast cancer, with 'early' covering all stages of the condition that have not spread to other organs, and 'late' for when there is spread to other parts of the body beyond the lymph nodes under the arm (the axillary nodes).

In Britain, the great majority of women will have early breast cancer when their condition is first diagnosed. Only about 1 in 20 women will have obvious secondary cancers in their bones or other organs when their breast cancer is discovered. Incidentally, another bit of medical jargon is 'presentation' – meaning the time a cancer is first found. So when doctors talk about these figures they might say: 'At presentation, 95 per cent of women have early breast cancer and 5 per cent have late breast cancer.'

Grading a breast cancer

There is no way of knowing for sure how fast any particular breast cancer will grow or how soon it will form secondary cancers in the lymph nodes or elsewhere. But one thing that does give doctors a clue about how a breast cancer might behave is the grade of the primary tumour.

When a breast cancer is removed the pathologist will look at it under a microscope and study the appearance of the cells that make up the cancer. Depending on what they see they will put the cancer into one of three grades.

Grade I cancer cells look quite similar to the normal cells in the breast and it is only when you look at them very carefully that you can see they are actually cancerous. Grade I cancers are also called well-differentiated cancers. In a grade III cancer the cells look nothing like breast cancer cells and they are very obviously malignant. Grade III cancers are also called poorly differentiated cancers. In a grade II breast cancer the appearance of the cells is somewhere between grades I and III; they are obviously abnormal but not that abnormal. Grade II cancers are also known as moderately differentiated cancers.

In general, grade III cancers will be more rapidly growing and likely to form secondary cancers sooner than grade II cancers. Grade I cancers will be slower growing and less likely to form metastases than grade II cancers. Another way of saying this is that grade III cancers tend to be more aggressive than grade II cancers and grade II cancers tend to be more aggressive than grade I cancers.

The grade of a cancer does not provide an absolute rule about how it will behave. Some grade III cancers will grow very slowly and be late to spread whereas some grade I cancers may grow quickly and spread early. But these will be the exceptions and, overall, the grade of a tumour is a useful guide to doctors in deciding how a breast cancer is likely to behave and what treatment to suggest.

Receptors

For over 100 years it has been known that changes in the level of the female hormone oestrogen in the bloodstream can affect the growth of some breast cancers. How this happens was not really understood until the 1950s, when the American scientist Elwood Jensen discovered oestrogen receptors. Oestrogen receptors are proteins in the cancer cell that collect oestrogen from the blood and take it to the cell nucleus. Once it is in the nucleus the oestrogen makes the cancer cell grow and produce new cancer cells.

Not all breast cancers are made up of cells with oestrogen receptors. Overall, about 3 out of 4 breast cancers have the receptors. The older you are the more likely it is that your breast cancer will have oestrogen receptors. These days all breast cancers are tested when they are first discovered to see whether or not they have oestrogen receptors. Those that do are called oestrogen receptor-positive and those that don't are oestrogen receptor-negative. Because oestrogen receptors were first discovered in the USA, and because Americans spell 'oestrogen' as 'estrogen' these cancers are known as either ER+ if they have the receptors and ER– if they don't.

When it comes to deciding treatment, knowing whether a breast cancer is ER+ or ER– is very important. If a tumour is ER+ then it is very likely to be sensitive to hormonal (endocrine) therapies; if it is ER– these treatments will not work and are a waste of time.

Another female hormone is called progesterone, and many breast cancers will carry receptors for this hormone as well. The presence or absence of progesterone receptors is much less important than the presence or absence of oestrogen receptors when it comes to

Hormones and the endocrine system

The endocrine system is a collection of glands in different parts of the body that produce hormones. These glands include the pituitary (in the head), the thyroid (in the neck) and the adrenals (one on top of each kidney). The testes and ovaries also act as endocrine glands, producing the male and female sex hormones (testosterone and oestrogen). The hormones themselves are chemicals that are released by the endocrine glands into the bloodstream, where they act as chemical messengers sending signals to other organs or tissues in the body.

In breast cancer treatment, if a tumour contains oestrogen receptors (if it is ER+) then giving treatment to reduce oestrogen levels or stop oestrogen from stimulating the cancer cells can be very important. This is generally called 'hormone therapy' or 'endocrine therapy'. Although these names are not strictly correct, because the drugs used are not hormones, they are acting to stop the effects of a particular hormone and so this has become the accepted way for doctors to talk about these treatments.

deciding treatment, so they are often not tested for. If the test is done and the receptors are present, the report will say that the breast cancer is PgR+; if they are not present it will be PgR–.

In the 1990s an entirely different type of receptor, called the HER2 receptor, was discovered in some breast cancers. This receptor is a protein that collects certain growth factors from the blood and combines with them to send signals to the cell nucleus telling it to grow and produce new cancer cells. Only about 1 in 3 breast cancers carry these receptors, but knowing if they are there or not is valuable when it comes to treatment as there are now a number of drugs available that can stop the receptor working and slow the growth of the cancer. Nowadays, all newly diagnosed breast cancers are tested to see whether or not they have the receptor. Those that do are called HER2+ and those that don't are called HER2–.

You

When it comes to deciding what is the best treatment for your breast cancer, knowing the size of the primary cancer and whether it is ER+ or ER– and HER2+ or HER2– (its receptor status), and knowing its stage and grade, are the most important factors. But your doctors will also need to take account of you, as well as your cancer, in making their recommendations. They will need to think about your age and your general fitness. Age is important because some treatments work better at different times of life than others or may cause more side effects at certain ages. Your general health is also important because some treatments may not be advisable if you have other illnesses or health problems.

It is also absolutely essential that your doctors also take account of your feelings about treatment. It is your cancer that is being treated and your body and mind that are going to have to cope with the effects of that treatment. The modern-day NHS insists that you are key to the decision-making process about your treatment, although how much opportunity you are actually given for this to happen varies enormously from doctor to doctor. But it is your right to ask all the questions you want to about any treatment that is recommended to you, and to get all the information you can before you decide whether or not to go ahead.

2

Treatment for breast cancer

The aim of this book is to explain how and why different types of treatment are used to cure breast cancer. In order to do this we first need to look at what those treatments actually are and what

The multidisciplinary team

You almost certainly won't meet the multidisciplinary team (MDT) during your hospital visits but you may hear people talk about it. The NHS introduced MDTs for breast cancer during the late 1990s. The idea behind MDTs was to bring together all the different experts who might be involved in a patient's care to discuss what the best approach to treatment might be. Before the creation of MDTs the various doctors involved in breast cancer care worked separately. The breast surgeon would read the report from a radiologist or pathologist and the oncologist would get letters from the surgeon and write back to them, but they would not get together and meet face to face to talk about the best way to manage any one woman's cancer. The feeling was that MDTs, where all the different doctors and the specialist nurses could meet and talk, would lead to a greater pooling of expertise, experience and knowledge, and better communication, which would lead to better decision-making. There was also a view that women would feel more confident if decisions about their treatment were made by a group of experts rather than a single individual. How much the introduction of MDTs has or has not improved the quality of treatment advice in breast cancer is still being debated, but at the present time any woman who has breast cancer diagnosed will have her case discussed by an MDT in order to plan her treatment.

Usually, the MDT makes fairly general recommendations. They might say that a woman needs surgery or radiotherapy or cytotoxic treatment, but it will then be the responsibility of the surgeon, the clinical oncologist or the medical oncologist to talk face to face with her and agree on the exact detail of which operation, the length of the course of radiation or which particular combination of drugs might be best in her situation.

words like 'radiotherapy' and 'chemotherapy' actually mean. In this chapter I am only going to talk about conventional treatment – the treatment you can expect from the NHS, which includes surgery, radiotherapy and drug treatment. There is a whole range of other therapies, both complementary and alternative, that women often turn to in order to help them cope with their cancer, and we will cover these in Chapter 10.

Surgery

Surgery is the oldest type of treatment for breast cancer, and it involves having an operation to take away the primary tumour in the breast. Up to about 1970 this almost always meant having a mastectomy – an operation to remove the breast.

In the first half of the twentieth century surgeons believed that the bigger the operation they did the more likely it was to lead to a cure. Consequently, by the 1950s the most widely used surgery for early breast cancer was a 'radical' mastectomy. This meant not only taking away the whole of the affected breast but also all the lymph nodes under the arm on that side of the body and the large muscles lying between the breast and the underlying ribs (the pectoral muscles).

Removing the muscles under the breast was very disfiguring. During the 1960s it was realized that the chance of a cure was just as good with a less drastic operation, without taking away those muscles, so long as radiotherapy was given after the surgery. This operation, where only the breast is removed, is called a 'simple' mastectomy.

As the idea of doing a simple mastectomy followed by radiotherapy became the norm, some surgeons wondered if they could do smaller operations and still get a cure. During the 1970s a number of large clinical trials showed that this was possible. Over time the operations became smaller and smaller. At first there was the partial mastectomy, where about half the breast was taken away, then the quadrantectomy, where the quarter of the breast with the cancer was removed, and then the lumpectomy, where just the cancer itself was taken away. A lumpectomy is also called a local excision or, if some of the surrounding normal breast tissue is also taken away, a wide local excision. With all these less extensive operations the clinical trials showed it was still necessary to give radiotherapy after the surgery to have the best chance of cure.

Just as the extent of surgery to the breast has tended to reduce over the last 40 years, so has the extent of surgery for the lymph nodes under the arm. It used to be thought that the surgeon should try and remove all the lymph nodes, an operation known as a total axillary clearance or axillary dissection. Then the idea of axillary sampling was introduced. This meant taking away four or five of the lymph nodes closest to the breast. If tests showed that the cancer had spread to those lymph nodes then the surgeon would usually go on to do an axillary clearance, taking away the remaining lymph nodes under the arm. But if the nodes were clear of any cancer either no further treatment would be given to the axilla or radiotherapy might be used as a precaution.

Over the last decade a further development has been the introduction of sentinel node biopsy. This involves having a special dye injected into the skin around the breast cancer an hour or two before it is due to be removed. When the surgeon does the operation to take away the breast cancer they can use the dye to trace the axillary lymph node nearest to the tumour – called the sentinel lymph node. They then remove the sentinel node, and if this is clear of any sign of cancer then it is almost certain that none of the other lymph nodes under the arm have been affected and so no further surgery is needed. If the gland does contain cancer then the surgeon will have do a further operation to clear the axillary nodes, or they may recommend a course of radiotherapy.

In the 1950s if a woman found she had a breast cancer she would be told the only surgical treatment was a radical mastectomy. Nowadays this operation is virtually never done and, as we have seen, there is a range of surgical alternatives. How breast surgeons choose which operation to recommend and how to decide what is right for you is something we will look at later.

Radiotherapy

Radiotherapy uses high-energy radiation, called ionizing radiation, to kill cancer cells. When radiotherapy is given after surgery for early breast cancer the machine that is almost always used is a linear accelerator (LinAc). LinAcs produce very high-energy beams of X-rays, which destroy cancer cells.

Radiotherapy, like surgery, is a local treatment that only affects a particular part of the body. This means that before you start the treatment there will be one or two visits to hospital for what are called planning sessions. These involve having special scans or X-rays of your breast and chest area and also having measurements taken of your size and shape. These sessions are usually run by a therapeutic radiographer – the health professional who will actually be doing your radiotherapy treatments. Sometimes you may be asked if the radiographer can make some small, permanent ink marks on your skin, which will help to make the treatment as accurate as possible. This is a bit like having a tattoo and just involves a small pin-prick for each mark – a small dot. Planning sessions usually last anywhere from half an hour to an hour and are always done as an outpatient.

The radiotherapy itself is a course of treatments all done as an outpatient. For each treatment you will have to undress your top half and put on a special gown. You then go into a large room and lie on a couch under the LinAc. The machine doesn't touch you during the treatment, and the treatment itself only takes a few minutes. Once you are on the couch the radiographers will take a

---

Who's who in your medical team?

General practitioner If you find a lump in your breast, or have other breast problems, then your GP (family doctor) will usually be the first doctor you see. If they feel there is any chance you may have a cancer they will make an appointment for you to be seen at the breast clinic at your nearest hospital (usually within 2 weeks). If you have a cancer that is found through breast screening you may not see your GP because the screening service will arrange your breast clinic appointment. However, the doctors at the breast clinic will write to your GP to keep them informed of what is going on.

Breast surgeon Your breast surgeon will be a consultant who specializes in diseases of the breast. Although cancer will form the major part of their work they will also deal with non-cancerous breast problems like cysts or benign tumours (most breast lumps are actually benign tumours or cysts, outnumbering cancers by about 4 to 1).

Specialist breast care nurse A nurse attached to the breast clinic team who is expert in helping and supporting women with breast problems, including cancer.

Clinical oncologist An oncologist is a doctor who specializes in the treatment of cancer. A clinical oncologist is a doctor who has been trained to give both radiotherapy and chemotherapy. So if you are going to have radiotherapy you will see a clinical oncologist. In some hospitals your clinical oncologist will also organize your drug treatment (if you need it) but in other hospitals you might see a medical oncologist for this part of your treatment. Clinical oncologists used to be called radiotherapists and some people still use this name.

Medical oncologist Medical oncologists are doctors who specialize in the drug treatment of cancer but do not give radiotherapy, so they will advise on cytotoxic treatment, hormone therapy and targeted drug therapy.

Therapeutic radiographers Your clinical oncologist will be in charge of your radiotherapy but your day-to-day treatment will be handled by therapeutic radiographers. You will be able to chat to them each day when you come for treatment and let them know if you have any problems or questions.

Chemotherapy nurses These are nurses who are specially trained to give chemotherapy treatment. They will see you before you start treatment to go over what is involved and answer any questions you have, and they will actually give your drug treatment at the hospital's chemotherapy clinic.

Radiologist These are the doctors who organize and analyse your X-rays and scans.

Pathologists These are the doctors who look at your biopsies and study your cancer when it is removed to give information about its size and grade, whether or not the lymph nodes are involved and whether the tumour has oestrogen or HER2 receptors.

bit of time to get you in the right position and check all the details of the treatment. They will then go out of the room to a nearby control room to start the treatment (they cannot be in the room with you during the treatment because of the radiation). Although they are not with you the radiographers will be watching you on a television screen so you can let them know if you have any problems during the treatment, in which case they will then stop the radiation and come in to help you.

Most treatment sessions involve having the radiation from at least two different directions. So you will have a treatment for a minute or two and then the LinAc will be switched off, the radiographers will come back in, and they will either move you or the LinAc to set up the second part of the radiation, which will take another couple of minutes. Normally, from the time you start to get undressed to the time you leave a treatment session takes about 20–30 minutes.

The treatments are usually given daily for 5 days a week, Monday to Friday. The total number of treatments is quite variable. Years ago it was common for 30 to 35 treatments to be given over 6 or 7 weeks. Over the past 10 years clinical trials have shown that shorter courses with as few as 15 treatments can be just as effective. At the moment these treatments are not standardized and the actual number you receive will depend on the custom and practice at your local radiotherapy unit, so your treatment may last anywhere from 3 to 6 weeks.

One other variable is the use of a boost dose. The radiotherapy treatment usually covers the whole of the breast from which the cancer has been removed (and occasionally the lymph nodes in the axilla). A boost dose is an extra treatment given only to that part of the breast where the cancer was located (rather than the whole breast). Clinical trials have been done to see how effective boost doses are in reducing the risk of the cancer coming back, but the results have not been very clear-cut. Because there is still uncertainty about how useful boost treatments are, some doctors recommend them whereas others do not.

The doctors who are in charge of your radiotherapy are called clinical oncologists. They are specialists who have been trained in both radiotherapy and the drug treatment of cancer.

Treatment with drugs

This is by far the most complicated part of breast cancer treatment, with a huge and ever increasing number of drugs being used. These drugs fall into four main groups: cytotoxic drugs, hormone therapies, targeted therapies and bisphosphonates.

Cytotoxic drugs

These are the drugs that most people think of as 'chemotherapy'. To doctors, chemotherapy means any kind of treatment involving drugs: taking paracetamol for a headache or antibiotics for an infection is chemotherapy. But to the media and most of the public, 'chemotherapy' is shorthand for the use of cytotoxic drugs to treat cancer.

Cytotoxic drugs first appeared immediately after the Second World War and more than 100 have been discovered over the last 65 years, many of which are used in treating breast cancer. They work by interfering with the process of cell division, which is how cancers grow. Unfortunately, there are lots of normal cells in the body that are constantly dividing in order to make new cells to replace those that have worn out and died. Cytotoxic drugs cannot tell the difference between cancer cells and normal cells, so dividing normal cells are damaged as well as cancer cells when these drugs are given. This means that cytotoxic drugs often cause a lot of side effects.

Although cytotoxic drugs work by attacking cell division, different drugs affect this process in different ways. This means that the damage done to cancer cells can be increased by combining several different cytotoxic drugs. This is certainly the case in breast cancer, where most of the cytotoxic treatments used involve two or more drugs being used together rather than giving a single drug. This is sometimes called combination chemotherapy.

When combination chemotherapy was first introduced in the 1960s it caused severe side effects because of the increased damage to normal cells. But doctors realized that normal cells recovered far more quickly than cancer cells from the injury caused by the drugs. They found that giving the treatment once every 3–4 weeks greatly reduced the severity of the side effects; so these days most cytotoxic treatments are given intermittently with intervals of a few weeks in between to allow normal cells to recover. Each of these episodes is called a cycle of treatment.

Most cytotoxic drugs have to be given as a drip into a vein (an infusion) but a few can be given as capsules or tablets. In early breast cancer, cytotoxic therapy usually involves four to eight cycles of treatment given over about 4–6 months.

Some of the cytotoxic drugs used in treating breast cancer include capecitabine, cisplatin, cyclophosphamide, docetaxel (Taxotere), doxorubicin, epirubicin, fluorouracil, methotrexate and paclitaxel (Taxol).

Drug names

The names by which drugs are known can be quite complicated and confusing. Apart from the fact that drugs often have strange or difficult-sounding names, most drugs also have two different names: their generic (or non-proprietary) name and their brand (or proprietary) name.

The generic name is the proper scientific name of a particular medicine whereas the brand name is the name under which the manufacturer sells it. For example, Herceptin is the brand name of the targeted drug with the generic name trastuzumab and Nolvadex is the brand name of a hormonal drug with the generic name of tamoxifen. The brand names of drugs are always written with a capital letter and generic names are always written with a lower-case letter.

Some drugs are better known by their brand names, like the hormonal therapy Arimidex (which has the generic name of anastrozole), and others are usually known by their generic name, like the cytotoxic drug epirubicin (which has the brand name Pharmorubicin).

In this book the first time a drug is mentioned I have used the generic name with the brand name in brackets afterwards.

Hormone therapies

We have already seen that most breast cancers carry oestrogen receptors (ER+ cancers). These tumours rely on the female hormone oestrogen, circulating in the bloodstream, to stimulate their growth. If your breast cancer is ER+ then hormone therapy can be very effective in helping to reduce the risk of it coming back after surgery. Incidentally, hormone therapy is often called endocrine therapy; hormone therapy and endocrine therapy are the same thing.

In younger women, who have not reached the menopause, the main source of oestrogen is the ovaries – the two small, walnut-sized organs that lie either side of the womb, in the pelvis. The release of oestrogen from the ovaries is controlled by other hormones, which are made by the pituitary gland, which lies under the brain behind the back of the nose. When women reach the menopause and their periods stop, the ovaries no longer make any oestrogen. But small amounts of oestrogen are still produced in the fatty tissues of the body. The key chemicals involved in this production are a group of enzymes called aromatases.

Hormone therapies work in one of two ways – either by reducing the amount of oestrogen in the bloodstream or by interfering with the oestrogen receptor so that the oestrogen can no longer bond to it.

In the early days, treatment to reduce oestrogen levels in younger women relied on surgery to remove either the ovaries (an oophorectomy) or the pituitary gland (a hypophysectomy). Nowadays drug treatment is almost always used. The drug most often given is called goserelin (Zoladex), which acts by switching off the pituitary hormones that tell the ovaries to release oestrogen. Zoladex is given as an injection under the skin of the abdomen once a month or once every 3 months. For women who are past the menopause there are a group of drugs that stop the aromatase enzymes from working and so stop fatty tissue producing the hormone. These drugs are called aromatase inhibitors and include anastrozole (Arimidex), letrozole (Femara) and exemestane (Aromasin). They are all given as tablets taken once a day.

The most commonly used drug that acts by interfering with the oestrogen receptor on breast cancer cells is tamoxifen. This binds

Timing of treatment

Surgery is the first part of any programme of breast cancer treatment, but if you also need radiotherapy and drug treatment the timing of these extra treatments varies. If you have decided to have chemotherapy with cytotoxic drugs then this usually starts as soon as you have recovered from surgery. The cytotoxic treatment will go on for between 4 and 6 months. If you need Herceptin (see page 32) then this is given after you finish cytotoxic treatment and can carry on for anywhere from 4 months to 2 years.

In the past, hormone treatment was started immediately after surgery and continued while you were having cytotoxic treatment and for some years after. But clinical trials showed that giving cytotoxic drugs and hormones at the same time actually made the treatment less effective. Because of these results the two types of treatment are no longer given together, so you may have hormone therapy for a brief period after your surgery, before you start cytotoxic treatment, but it will be stopped once you start your chemotherapy and you will be given the hormone treatment again once the cytotoxic drugs have finished. Hormone therapy and Herceptin can be given at the same time, as can hormone therapy and radiotherapy, without any loss of effectiveness. So if you need Herceptin or radiotherapy then your hormone treatment can carry on at the same time.

The timing of radiotherapy is variable. It can be given at the same time as cytotoxic or hormonal therapy, but many oncologists feel that giving radiotherapy along with cytotoxic drugs increases the risk of tiredness and other side effects and so they delay radiotherapy until cytotoxic treatment has finished. But other oncologists believe that their patients would prefer to get treatment over and done with as soon as possible and won't mind feeling a bit more tired if it means they can get things done more quickly. From a strictly medical point of view there is no need to give radiotherapy sooner rather than later, so the timing of this part of your treatment is something you can discuss with your oncologist and choose the timetable that you prefer.

to the receptor and stops oestrogen from attaching to it. Because it works by attaching to the receptor, rather than by reducing the oestrogen level in the bloodstream, tamoxifen is effective for both younger (premenopausal) and older (postmenopausal) women; the aromatase inhibitors only work for those women who are past the menopause. Tamoxifen is given as a tablet and is taken once a day.

Until very recently, hormonal treatments used as part of the treatment of early breast cancer were given for 5 years, but in the last few years some clinical trials have suggested that longer periods of treatment may sometimes give better results.

Targeted therapies

These drugs are newer than the cytotoxic drugs and hormone therapies and first began to appear during the 1990s. There is still no universal agreement over what they should be called, so some people talk about them as biological therapies or (incorrectly) as immunological therapies.

Many normal cells in our bodies are constantly dividing and multiplying. This cell division is controlled by proteins called growth factors, which circulate in the blood and bind to receptors on the surface of cells. This binding of the growth factor and receptor sends signals to the cell's nucleus that tell the cell to divide. Over the last 20 years a number of different growth factor receptors have been discovered. What has also been discovered is that in some cancers the cells make too many of these receptors, which means they are over-sensitive to the growth factors in the blood. This makes them multiply more than they should.

These discoveries have led scientists to look for drugs that can interfere with the growth factor receptors in the hope that these might be effective treatments for cancer. Many such drugs have been developed over the last 20 years and have formed an entirely new type of cancer treatment. A key difference between these drugs and the older cytotoxic drugs is that they only attack those cells producing too much of the receptor. In other words they only attack cancer cells and not normal cells. This is why they are called targeted therapies, because they target cancer cells while sparing normal cells. This means they tend to have fewer side effects than cytotoxic drugs, although they do still have some side effects of their own.

The growth factor receptor that has been most important so far in breast cancer is called HER2 (which is short for human epithelial growth factor receptor 2). A number of drugs have now been developed that target this receptor. The first and most widely used of these was trastuzumab (Herceptin). More recently developed drugs targeting the HER2 receptor include lapatinib (Tyverb) and pertuzumab (Omnitarg).

Only about 1 in 3 breast cancers actually makes too much HER2. This means that only about 1 in 3 breast cancers will be sensitive to treatment with Herceptin and the other HER2 targeted drugs. So for most women with breast cancer Herceptin and similar drugs won't be of any help.

Another receptor that has been shown to be important in some breast cancers is called VEGFR (which stands for vascular endothelial growth factor receptor) and a drug called bevacizumab (Avastin), which targets this receptor, has been tested in women with advanced breast cancer.

Research into growth factor receptors has been, and continues to be, a major area of cancer research over the last two decades, and more receptors, and more drugs to target those receptors, will undoubtedly be found in the years to come.

Bisphosphonates

The bisphosphonates are a group of drugs that build up the strength of the bones. They are sometimes used as part of the treatment for osteoporosis – the thinning and weakening of the bones that can sometimes happen in later life.

The bisphosphonates are regularly used in the treatment of women with advanced breast cancer when it has spread to their bones. They reduce the risk of the bones breaking (fractures) and also help with easing the pain that bone secondaries often cause.

In recent years doctors have wondered if giving bisphosphonates to women with early breast cancer would stop bone secondaries developing and improve the chance of a cure. Clinical trials are still looking at this question but the results so far have not shown a benefit from giving bisphosphonates – the number of women whose breast cancer spread to their bones was similar, whether or not they were given the drugs. So for the time being, if you have early breast cancer you are only likely to be offered treatment with bisphosphonates as part of a clinical trial.

3

How can breast cancer be cured?

The aim of treatment for breast cancer is to get rid of it and make sure it never comes back. When a cancer does come back, doctors call this a recurrence or a relapse. So the aim of treatment is to make sure there is never a relapse or a recurrence; in other words the aim of treatment is to get a cure. But what is 'a cure', how do you get it and how do you know whether you have got it or not? These are the questions we'll explore in this chapter.

What is a cure?

From the time when records first began to be kept in the mid 1920s until the mid 1970s, the cure rate for breast cancer in the UK and the USA did not change; it stuck stubbornly at about 50 per cent. Half of the women who developed the disease were cured but half died from their breast cancer. The pattern remained depressingly similar throughout this time. Women had a mastectomy and radiotherapy, which seemed to get rid of their cancer, but within a year or two half of them had developed secondary breast cancer (spread of their cancer to other parts of their body) and despite attempts at treatment, which might briefly slow the progress of their illness, they eventually died. Just getting rid of the primary breast cancer did not guarantee a cure. There was always the chance, and in those days it was a 50:50 chance, that the cancer would come back. Just to reassure you, the chances of a cure are far greater today, with more than 8 out of 10 women being cured, and the results are getting better all the time.

If the cancer could come back, how would you know when everything was clear – when you were cured? To this day there is still no scan, no X-ray, no blood test that can say whether or not someone is cured of breast cancer (or any other cancer). At the end of treatment women very often ask if there is a test they can have to see if they are safe and their cancer has gone forever. Unfortunately, the answer is no, no such test exists. The only way of knowing if you are cured or not is the passage of time. But how long do you have to wait before you can be sure your cancer will never come back?

The first attempts to answer this question were made over 50 years ago at the Christie Hospital in Manchester. Doctors looked at the records of people who had been treated for cancers of the mouth and throat and discovered that if they were still alive 5 years after their treatment, with no sign of cancer, their cancers never came back – they were cured. This work led to a widespread belief that anyone who had cancer, had treatment and was free of that cancer 5 years later, was cured.

Over time it was realized that in many types of cancer, including breast cancer, the disease could come back and secondary cancers could appear more than 5 years after the first treatment had been given. Medical statisticians went back to the drawing board and after a lot of research came up with a truer but much more complicated definition of a cure. They said that for any particular type of cancer (breast cancer, lung cancer, bowel cancer or whatever), the condition was cured when the survival of people with that cancer became the same as people of the same age and sex who did not have the cancer.

While this definition of cure has worked well in other cancers, there is a problem in breast cancer. Even 30 years after treatment the survival of women with breast cancer and other women is not quite the same. In other words even after 30 years breast cancer can sometimes come back. This is very, very rare but it has happened, and has led some experts to say that you can never be certain a breast cancer has been cured. In a strictly scientific, statistical sense this may be true but in the real world most relapses, most recurrences of the cancer, happen in the first 5 years after treatment, and the chances of your cancer coming back after 10 years are very small indeed. So if 5 years after treatment there is no sign of cancer then your chance of cure is very good, and if all is well and clear after 10 years then you are almost certainly cured.

Why does breast cancer come back?

If it isn't cured when it is first treated, why does breast cancer come back? The short answer to this is because it never actually went away.

The first line of treatment for early breast cancer gets rid of the primary tumour in the breast. When a relapse occurs, when the cancer 'comes back', it reappears not as another cancer in the breast but as secondary cancers, metastases, in other parts of the body: the bones, liver, lungs or brain or in lymph nodes other than those under the arm. These secondary cancers will have spread from the primary cancer in the breast. But they must have been there *before* that primary cancer was taken away. They cannot be spread to other places from a cancer that your surgeon has already operated on and removed.

If the secondary cancers were there when you had your initial operation, why were they not obvious, why were they not causing symptoms, why can your doctors not find them and treat them? The answer is because they were too small. Cancer cells are microscopic. A cancer the size of a pea contains more than 100 million cells, almost twice as many cells as there are people in Britain. So each individual cancer cell is unbelievably tiny.

Secondary cancers are made when small clumps of cells break away from the primary cancer and are carried off by the bloodstream or the lymph vessels. These small clumps may be made up of no more than a few tens or hundreds of cells. These little islands of cells come to rest somewhere else, in a distant lymph gland or in a bone or some other organ of the body. They set up home there and in so doing have made a secondary cancer. But that secondary cancer will be far too small to be seen by the naked eye, far too small to be picked up by any medical test and far too small to cause any symptoms or problems.

But the cells in that metastasis are cancer cells. That means they will divide and multiply. Over time that metastasis, that secondary cancer, will grow. Different cancers grow at different rates but eventually the metastasis will be big enough to start to cause symptoms – it may appear as a lump, be painful, make you feel sick or breathless, or give you a headache, depending on where it is, but it will let you know that something is wrong. It may take only a few months for this to happen or it may take several years, but when it does happen, when the secondary cancer is diagnosed, then that is when the cancer has relapsed. The cancer has 'come back' but actually it never went away – it was just that the minute seedlings of breast cancer cells that had already travelled to other places away from the breast, before you had your lumpectomy or mastectomy, were too small to be found, too small to cause any problems.

It took doctors a very long time to realize this. For the first half of the twentieth century they thought the key to treating breast cancer was to do bigger and bigger operations, taking away not only the breast but as much of the tissue around it as they possibly could. But although the surgery got more and more heroic, the operations more and more mutilating and distressing, the cure rate did not change. It was only when doctors began to realize that the real problem was those microscopic seedlings of cancer that had already escaped from the breast to other parts of the body that the way breast cancer was treated began to change, a change that has led to the huge improvement in the chance of cure that we see today.

The 1970s: a new understanding of breast cancer and its treatment

Until the 1970s 1 in every 2 women who had breast cancer died from their illness. These women died not from a lump in their breast, their primary breast cancer, but from the effects of the secondary cancers that had come from that primary cancer and gone to other parts of their bodies. As we have seen, those secondary cancers were made by invisible seedlings of clusters of cancer cells that had broken away from the primary breast cancer and escaped to the bones, the liver, the lungs or elsewhere before the surgeon had taken away that primary cancer. By the 1970s doctors realized that if they were going to improve the chance of a cure for women with breast cancer, they had to find a way of dealing with those potentially lethal but invisible seedlings of secondary cancer. Doing bigger and bigger operations to take away the primary cancer was not the answer.

Because they were too small to be seen there was no way of knowing where these tiny secondary cancers might be (or even if they were there at all), so doing an operation to remove them was impossible. The only way of dealing with them would be to give a drug or drugs that would get into the bloodstream and go to all parts of the body, killing cancer cells wherever they were hiding.

The change in thinking about breast cancer treatment, the realization that surgery alone was not enough for many women and that some type of drug therapy was also needed, came at just the right time. Until the 1970s drug treatment for breast cancer had been very limited; only a handful of drugs existed that had any effect and these often gave little real benefit. But at the end of the 1960s tamoxifen became available, which was a major advance in the hormone treatment of breast cancer. At the same time clinical trials were showing very encouraging results from giving combination cytotoxic chemotherapy to women who had advanced, metastatic, breast cancer. Although the use of these treatments did not actually lead to any cures of advanced breast cancer, they did often bring about dramatic reductions in the extent of the disease, shrinkage of the secondary cancers and relief of painful or distressing symptoms. They also increased life expectancy – women with advanced breast cancer were living longer as a result of these new drug treatments.

A trio of pioneering breast surgeons, Bernard Fisher in the USA, Gianni Bonadonna in Italy and Roar Nissen-Meyer in Norway, put together these two developments in breast cancer – the realization that microscopic secondary cancers were the cause of the disease coming back and that new drugs could shrink large measurable metastases in advanced breast cancer. They suggested that giving those same drugs to women with early breast cancer, after their primary breast cancer had been removed, might do more than just shrink any microscopic secondary cancers and might actually kill them off completely and bring about a cure. So they set about doing clinical trials, which very quickly showed that adding drug treatment to surgery in early breast cancer dramatically increased the chance of a cure.

Those clinical trials opened the way to the modern-day treatment of early breast cancer and pioneered the use of drug treatment to improve the chance of cure. The idea of giving drugs after surgery to reduce the chance of cancer coming back, by killing microscopic traces of the disease that have spread to other parts of the body, has become known as adjuvant therapy. This has become an important part of the treatment of many other cancers as well as breast cancer.

Neo-adjuvant chemotherapy

When women have cytotoxic chemotherapy or other drugs as part of their treatment for early breast cancer, this is called adjuvant therapy. Adjuvant therapy is usually given after surgery has been carried out to remove the primary breast cancer.

Occasionally, cytotoxic chemotherapy is actually given before surgery. This may sometimes be done to try and shrink a large primary cancer to make an operation easier. It is also done in an uncommon condition called inflammatory breast cancer, where the cancer spreads through the fine lymph vessels throughout the breast, making the whole breast appear swollen, red and inflamed. When cytotoxic chemotherapy is given before a mastectomy or a lumpectomy it is called neo-adjuvant chemotherapy.

As a result of the use of adjuvant drug therapy the likelihood of a cure for women with early breast cancer has risen from around 50 per cent to over 80 per cent and is still rising, so that now more than 8 out of every 10 women with early breast cancer are likely to have treatment that will mean their cancer never comes back. But this does lead to two vital questions for anyone who has early breast cancer: do I need drug treatment as well as surgery and, if I do, what drugs should I have? These are questions we will look at in the coming chapters.

4

Surgery: your first treatment choice

Surgery remains the cornerstone of treatment for early breast cancer. When a breast cancer is suspected, either because you have found a lump or have had an abnormal mammogram from breast screening, you will be given an appointment at your local breast clinic. These hospital-based clinics are run by surgeons who specialize in the treatment of breast cancer. They will be supported by a team of nurses who are experts in the care and support of women with breast cancer (specialist breast nurses) and more junior doctors who are training to be experts in the field (see pages 21 and 24–5).

Triple assessment

At the breast clinic the first thing to find out is whether or not you do have a breast cancer; this involves what has become known as a triple assessment. The triple assessment is made up of an examination of your breasts, radiology (imaging) of your breast, and a biopsy. Radiology will usually mean having a mammogram (a breast X-ray) but may also include an ultrasound scan of your breasts (this is quite painless and involves having a sort of microphone gently rubbed over the skin of your breasts for a few minutes to produce sound pictures of the underlying tissue). A biopsy is usually done with a needle and takes away a small sample of tissue from your breast. This sample can be examined under the microscope to see if there is any sign of cancer.

The examination of your breasts will look for the size and position of any lumps in your breasts and also check to see whether or not there are any obviously enlarged lymph nodes under your arm. If you have DCIS (ductal carcinoma *in situ*; see Chapter 1) there is often no lump to feel and the changes only show up on a mammogram or ultrasound examination. So having a mammogram (and possibly an ultrasound scan as well) will give more information about the size and position of any suspicious lump in your breast and will also help detect DCIS. The biopsy will show whether your lump, or any suspicious area shown by the radiology, is cancerous or not. The biopsy will also give other very important information, including whether the cancer is DCIS or an invasive breast cancer (see Chapter 1). It will also give the grade of the tumour and whether or not it has oestrogen receptors (ER+ or ER–) or HER2 receptors (HER2+ or HER2–).

With the information from the radiology and the biopsy, and the examination findings, your surgeon will then be able to talk to you about the first stage in your treatment and what that might be. The advice they give will depend on whether you have DCIS or an invasive breast cancer.

Surgery for DCIS

DCIS used to be very infrequently diagnosed but that changed with the introduction of breast screening in the UK during the 1980s. Since then there has been a tenfold increase in the number of DCIS diagnosed, and about 1 in every 5 cancers discovered by breast screening will be DCIS.

DCIS remains a rather mysterious condition because although it will very often change into an invasive breast cancer if it is not treated (although this may take as long as 10–15 years), it is clear that sometimes it never develops into an invasive cancer and even if nothing is done will never cause any problems. Unfortunately, at the present time there is no test that can be done to say whether a DCIS will turn into an invasive cancer at some time in the future or whether it is essentially harmless and can be left alone.

In the last few years some experts have argued that because DCIS may be harmless, and as this is more likely with smaller tumours and those that have a low grade, then for some women giving no immediate treatment and simply doing regular follow-up examinations and radiology may be all that's needed. This is a controversial suggestion and the great majority of breast surgeons still think DCIS should always be treated. Certainly, when I have talked about this with women at my Breast Cancer Care meetings they have always said they would want something done rather than having to live with the thought that there was something in their breast that could become a cancer. But if you are absolutely determined that you want to avoid surgery if at all possible then discussing with your breast surgeon the question of regular follow-up as an alternative may be an option.

For many years the usual treatment for DCIS was a mastectomy. This is still an option and will almost always lead to a cure – only about 2 out of every 100 women will have any recurrence of their cancer after a mastectomy. Studies have shown that having a smaller operation (a lumpectomy), taking away only the DCIS and leaving the rest of the breast intact, is just as good at getting a cure as a mastectomy if it is followed by radiotherapy to the remaining breast tissue. But these figures do relate to long-term cure – among women who opt for a lumpectomy and radiotherapy about 1 in 10 will develop a recurrence of their cancer in the breast and need a mastectomy in order to gain their cure.

Usually you will have a choice between a mastectomy or a lumpectomy, but sometimes your surgeon will advise that a mastectomy is essential. This is likely if the area of DCIS in your breast is quite large, about 5 cm or more across, or if there is more than one area of DCIS in different parts of the breast (doctors call this a multifocal cancer). If you have very small breasts your surgeon may also suggest that the cosmetic result following surgery may be better if you have a mastectomy.

In deciding whether to have a mastectomy or a lumpectomy and radiotherapy, different women have very different priorities. Some feel that if there is anything wrong with the breast they just want it all taken away so that they can have peace of mind and don't have to worry about the cancer coming back. For other women, keeping their breast, or as much of it as possible, is all important and they would feel very damaged if they had to have a mastectomy. Only you know how you feel about your breasts and so this is very much your decision.

If you decide on the lumpectomy and radiotherapy option, remember that this does mean there is about a 1 in 10 chance that sometime during the next 10–15 years the cancer will come back and you will need a mastectomy. There is no way of telling for sure how likely this is but the risk is greater in younger women (under the age of 45 years), in those women who have an actual lump in the breast (rather than the DCIS having been picked up by a screening mammogram) and if the DCIS is high grade (grade III). So if one or more of these applies to you, you may feel more inclined towards a mastectomy but equally you may prefer to go for the lumpectomy and radiotherapy since the chances of a complete cure are still about 90 per cent with this approach.

Because DCIS very rarely spreads beyond the breast you won't usually need any surgery to the lymph nodes under your arm and normally the only treatment choice you will have to make about surgery is whether to go for a mastectomy or a lumpectomy and radiotherapy. Unless you have a large area of DCIS or a multifocal tumour then the choice is yours.

Surgery for invasive breast cancer

The breast

The aim of surgery is to remove your primary breast cancer completely. Mastectomy is an option but so are less major operations; these are talked about as breast-sparing operations, breast-conserving operations or conservative surgery. The most common of these conservative operations is a lumpectomy, where just the cancer and a small margin of normal tissue around it are removed. An alternative is a quadrantectomy, where the cancer is taken away together with about a quarter of the breast that surrounds it.

As with DCIS, the choice between mastectomy or a conservative operation is usually down to you. If your primary breast cancer is more than 5 cm across or if there is more than one cancer in the breast (which is more usually an area of DCIS but very occasionally two invasive cancers can occur in the same breast at the same time) then a mastectomy will usually be necessary and it would not be safe to have a less extensive operation.

If you have a mastectomy then you often won't need to have radiotherapy following your surgery, although this is occasionally necessary (see pages 53–4). If you have a lumpectomy or quadrantectomy then radiotherapy is almost always essential to minimize the risk of cancer coming back in the remaining breast tissue. The chance of a cure will be the same whether you have a mastectomy or a more conservative operation followed by radiotherapy, so the choice of surgery really is down to you and what you would like.

One thing that might influence your decision is the possibility of breast reconstruction after a mastectomy. Breast reconstruction aims to give you back a normal breast shape after surgery, and there are a number of different operations that can be done. The reconstruction may involve inserting a prosthesis (an artificial breast) between the skin and the underlying muscle on the chest, or replacing the lost breast tissue with skin, fat or muscle from somewhere else in your body, or it may use a combination of these two approaches. The type of operation that might be recommended depends on your body shape, your general fitness and your age. It will also be influenced by the experience of your surgeon and the operations that they feel give the best results.

Breast reconstruction doesn't give you back a normal breast and it is important to ask to see photographs of other women who have had the operation and ideally to talk to someone who has had the surgery so that you can get an idea of what the results are like before you make a decision. Other things to bear in mind are that your new breast will feel different and won't have the same sensitivity as a normal breast, and may actually be numb. Breast reconstruction also usually involves more than one operation in a matter of some weeks or even months and may involve having to travel to another hospital some distance away. If the reconstruction involves taking tissue from other parts of your body, this will leave scars and possibly some discomfort. There are also all the normal possible complications of any operation to think about, like infection or delayed wound healing. On the more positive side, having a reconstruction will mean you won't have to wear a breast prosthesis to give you a breast shape. When you are dressed you will have the same appearance as you did before your mastectomy and you will also have a cleavage and be able to wear low neckline clothes. Having a breast reconstruction won't increase the risk of cancer coming back and won't make check-ups for cancer any more difficult.

Breast reconstruction may be available as an option at the time you have your mastectomy or it may only be possible some months later. This varies from hospital to hospital. A detailed discussion of the different types of operation you can have is beyond the scope of this book, but Breast Cancer Care (see 'Useful addresses' at the end of the book) has an excellent free booklet, *Breast Reconstruction*, which has all this information and other useful advice to help you make up your mind. If you decide not to have a reconstruction then Breast Cancer Care also has another booklet, *A Confident Choice: Breast Prostheses, Bras and Clothes After Surgery*, that you might find very helpful.

The axilla

Surgery to the lymph nodes under the arm next to the breast in which the primary tumour is located has two aims: first to get rid of any cancer that might have spread to those lymph nodes and second to stage the cancer (to see how far it has spread), which will help in deciding what further treatment, if any, may be needed.

As late as the 1990s the approach to treatment of the axillary nodes was very aggressive and usually involved an operation to take away the glands (an axillary clearance, or axillary dissection), followed by a course of radiotherapy to the area under the arm. This gets rid of any cancer in the glands but can lead to severe side effects. The main one of these is lymphoedema. Lymphoedema is swelling of the arm, which may appear days, months or occasionally years after treatment to the axilla. With axillary clearance alone, or radiotherapy to the axilla alone, about 1 in 5 women will develop lymphoedema. When the two treatments are combined this figure can rise to as high as 1 out of 2 women being affected.

Lymphoedema varies hugely in its severity. It may be no more than a very slight swelling of the arm that can only be detected by careful measurement, but at the other end of the scale it can cause massive swelling, gross disfigurement and severe disability, making the arm virtually useless and very painful. Although a lot can be done to help control and reduce lymphoedema if it occurs, there is no cure – no way of putting back the missing lymph nodes and lymph vessels in the axilla, the loss of which has stopped effective drainage of lymph from the arm and leads to the swelling. Recognizing this, and recognizing the distress that lymphoedema can cause has led doctors to change their way of treating the axilla.

The approach that the National Institute for Health and Clinical Excellence (NICE) recommends in its guidance on early breast cancer, which is followed by most breast clinics, is to do an ultrasound examination of the axilla before breast surgery. If the ultrasound scan shows any apparently suspicious, enlarged or abnormal lymph nodes then the next step is to do a needle biopsy, which can be done as an outpatient with a local anaesthetic (so it may be a bit uncomfortable but should not be painful). If the biopsy shows evidence of cancer then an axillary clearance to remove all the lymph nodes is recommended. This would not usually be followed by radiotherapy so there would be about a 1 in 5 risk of lymphoedema, but this would be offset by the improved chance of cure resulting from removal of the nodes.

NICE

The National Institute for Health and Clinical Excellence (NICE) was set up by the NHS in 1999 to try and reduce differences in the quality of treatment across the country – the so-called 'postcode lottery'. It uses groups of independent experts to report on the effectiveness and value for money of treatments and to produce guidelines as to how different cancers (and many other illnesses) should be treated.

Each of these expert teams includes patient representatives. All NICE's reports are available online at <http://www.nice.org.uk> and all have patient-friendly versions. The latest general guides that NICE has produced on breast cancer were both published in 2009: *Early and Locally Advanced Breast Cancer: Diagnosis and Treatment*, NICE clinical guideline 80 (download at <http://www.nice.org.uk/CG80>) and *Advanced Breast Cancer: Diagnosis and Treatment*, NICE clinical guideline 81 (download at <http://www.nice.org.uk/CG81>). NICE also produces what it calls technical reports, which assess new treatments for cancer as and when they become available. These reports are also available online.

For those women who have a normal axillary ultrasound scan, or who have a needle biopsy that shows no sign of cancer, then the next step is a sentinel node biopsy (see page 23). If the sentinel node biopsy is clear, with no sign of cancer, then no further surgery is needed. If the biopsy is positive, with cancer in the gland, then an axillary clearance is needed to get rid of any further cancer and to stage the disease accurately. This is the current national guidance but recent clinical trials have suggested that if the sentinel lymph node biopsy is positive, showing signs of cancer, then provided that chemotherapy is given there is no need for an axillary clearance as the chance of cure is just as good. This means that some breast surgeons might suggest that you won't need an operation to take away your axillary lymph nodes if you are going to have chemotherapy. However, many will feel that they need to see evidence from more clinical trials before they can make this recommendation with confidence.

Sentinel node biopsy is still a relatively new procedure and there are still some breast clinics in the UK where it is not available; in these hospitals axillary node sampling offers an alternative. This is where the surgeon operates on the axilla but only removes the three or four nodes closest to the breast to be checked to see if any cancer is present. This carries a very small risk of lymphoedema but much less than with a full axillary clearance.

What if I do nothing?

Having surgery or not having surgery is your choice. It is the single most important choice you can make in hoping to get a cure from your cancer. Many women with breast cancer are cured just by having an operation. If you don't have surgery to take away your primary cancer then you almost certainly will not be cured. If you are over the age of 80 years and have a small cancer that is ER+ then it is just possible that treatment with hormone drugs and radiotherapy will keep your cancer in check and allow you to lead a normal life. But for younger women, leaving their primary cancer alone will eventually be a fatal decision. Different breast cancers grow at very different speeds: sometimes it will be years before they spread to form distant secondary cancers, but often it is only a matter of a few months or a year or so and then, whatever is done, it is too late to get a cure; treatment may prolong life but will never completely get rid of the cancer.

When it comes to deciding whether or not to have an operation to take away your primary breast cancer you have, in reality, no choice and you should always go for the operation. Once you have made that decision you can then talk with your surgeon and breast care nurse, your GP, your family and friends and whoever else you think can help, and decide exactly what your options are and what type of surgery you would like to go for.

5

Radiotherapy

Radiotherapy, like surgery, is a local treatment and will only affect that part of the body which is irradiated. When radiotherapy is given after surgery for early breast cancer, the aim is to reduce the risk of cancer coming back in the remaining breast tissue (after a lumpectomy) or in the skin overlying the front of the chest (after a mastectomy). Giving radiotherapy to the breast or chest area will not have any effect on microscopic secondary cancers anywhere else in the body. Occasionally, radiotherapy will also be given to the axilla, the area under the arm. Much less often radiotherapy will also be given to the area above the collarbone (the supraclavicular area) on the same side of the body, to irradiate the supraclavicular lymph nodes that lie under the skin in that region.

Radiotherapy after conservative surgery

After a primary breast cancer has been taken away by a breast-sparing operation like a lumpectomy or quadrantectomy, most of the breast will still be left and there is a danger that the cancer could come back in that breast tissue. This might happen if microscopic clusters of cancer cells were left behind after the operation that could grow back to form another cancerous breast lump in the future.

In 1976 a large clinical trial was started in the USA where women with early breast cancer were treated either with a lumpectomy alone, a lumpectomy followed by radiotherapy to the remaining breast tissue or a mastectomy. Twenty-five years later the results of the study showed that of every 100 women who had a lumpectomy with no radiotherapy, 39 developed a recurrence of their cancer in the same breast. In the women who had a lumpectomy and radiotherapy, only 14 out of every 100 had their cancer come back in the same breast. Very obviously, having radiotherapy after a lumpectomy greatly reduced the risk of the cancer coming back in the same breast: from almost a 40 per cent chance to a less than 15 per cent chance.

But that same study also showed that the chance of cure was the same whether or not women had radiotherapy after their lumpectomy. This is because if a cancer comes back in the breast after a lumpectomy it is almost always possible to do a mastectomy to take away the recurrent cancer and the remaining breast tissue. Surgeons often call this a 'salvage' mastectomy. After a salvage mastectomy, between half and two-thirds of women with a recurrent cancer will be cured. (The reason not all women are cured is because some will develop secondary cancers in other parts of their body, and removing their breast will have no effect in preventing these growing.)

It is now routine practice for doctors to recommend for most women a course of radiotherapy to the remaining breast tissue after a lumpectomy or quadrantectomy. There is some debate among breast cancer experts as to whether this is necessary in older women over the age of 70 years who have cancers that have not spread to the lymph nodes under the arm and whose cancers are ER+. Clinical trials have suggested that giving hormone therapy after a lumpectomy in these women may be just as effective as radiotherapy in preventing cancer coming back in their breast.

In the past, having radiotherapy after surgery for breast cancer often involved treatment 5 days a week, Monday to Friday, for 6 or 7 weeks (30 to 35 treatments). Clinical trials have now shown that much shorter courses with as few as 15 treatments over 3 weeks are just as effective in preventing cancer coming back in the breast. However, there is still a lot of variation between different oncologists: some will recommend 15 treatments, others will advise 20, 25 or even 30 treatments. It is difficult to explain these differences because there is no medical evidence to show that longer courses of treatment are any better. Some doctors use the longer treatments because that was the way they were trained and what they are used to; others believe the longer treatments cause fewer side effects and give better cosmetic results, even though clinical trials have never shown this to be the case.

Another variable is boost radiotherapy: giving a short extra course of treatment (anywhere from one to ten treatments but usually five) to that part of the breast from which the cancer was removed. The hope is that this will further reduce the risk of the cancer coming back but it also increases the risk of side effects and a worse cosmetic result as well as adding extra hospital visits. Clinical trials have not given clear answers for or against giving boost radiotherapy, and current guidelines suggest that it should only be used if there is a high risk of the cancer coming back. But oncologists vary in their opinions about boost treatment – some advise it for almost everyone whereas others are very sparing and only suggest it if they are really concerned the cancer could come back.

Radiotherapy after a mastectomy

The clinical trial in the USA that I mentioned in the previous section showed that about 1 in 10 of those women who were treated by a mastectomy developed a recurrence of their cancer in the skin where the breast had been removed. Other studies have shown that this figure can be reduced by giving radiotherapy to the skin overlying the front of the chest on that side after a mastectomy. But as 9 out 10 women don't need this treatment, research has been done to see if it is possible to work out who is more likely to be at risk of developing a recurrence and only offering radiotherapy to those women.

Among the factors that have been found to increase the chances of cancer coming back in the skin after a mastectomy are:

- a large primary cancer, more than 5 cm across;
- a primary cancer that has spread to the lymph nodes under the arm;
- a high grade (grade III) primary cancer;
- a primary cancer that has no oestrogen receptors (ER–);
- breast cancer in younger women under the age of 40 years.

Although these risk factors have been worked out, there is no agreement how to use them to advise women about treatment. Some oncologists will say that if a woman has any one of these risks she should have radiotherapy after her mastectomy; others only advise radiation if there are two risk factors and others only if three or more are present.

If no radiotherapy is given after a mastectomy and months or years later a local recurrence of the cancer does appear in the skin on the chest wall then this can be treated by an operation followed by radiotherapy. The evidence from clinical trials suggests that the chance of cure is as good in this situation as if radiotherapy had been given at the time of the original surgery.

Once again, the number of radiotherapy treatments that might be recommended after a mastectomy is very variable and can range from 15 in 3 weeks to 30 or 35 in 6–7 weeks. But a boost dose is not used in this situation.

Radiotherapy to the lymph nodes under the arm

The aim of treating the lymph nodes in the axilla next to the breast is to kill off any traces of cancer that might be in those glands and go on to spread to other parts of the body or continue to grow there causing swelling and pain.

In the past, treatment of these glands was very aggressive and meant surgery to take them away (an axillary clearance) followed by high-dose radiotherapy. But this very often led to the complication of lymphoedema – swelling and discomfort in the arm on that side of the body, which can often be very distressing (see page 46). There was also the risk of a much less common but very severe side effect: brachial nerve damage. The brachial nerves are the nerves that make the arm work, controlling all its movements and carrying all sense of feeling from the arm. Injury to the brachial nerves can leave the arm paralysed and numb: a completely useless arm. The brachial nerves lie very close to the lymph nodes in the axilla and, in the past, well-meaning but over-aggressive treatment of the nodes sometimes led to severe and irreversible damage to those nerves, with disastrous consequences.

Because of the risk of lymphoedema and brachial nerve damage, radiotherapy to the axilla is used much less often these days. If neither a sentinel node biopsy nor axillary sampling show any sign of cancer in the lymph nodes then there is no need for radiotherapy. If sentinel node biopsy or axillary sampling have shown signs of cancer, and surgery with an axillary clearance has then been done, then once again there is no need for radio-therapy. This means that radiation of the axillary lymph nodes is only needed if a sentinel node biopsy or axillary sampling has shown signs of cancer in the lymph glands but for some reason surgery to remove the remaining glands under the arm is not possible. The net result of all this is that these days most women with early breast cancer will not need to have radiotherapy to their axilla.

Radiotherapy to the supraclavicular lymph nodes

When breast cancer cells are carried away from a primary breast cancer by the bloodstream they can travel all over the body; there is no pattern to where the cells might go and where secondary cancers might develop. But when the cancer cells move through the lymph vessels the process is usually much more orderly, the sentinel lymph node being the first to be affected and then the remaining glands under the arm. From these axillary lymph nodes the next stage on the journey is to the glands that lie above the armpit, above and behind the collar bone (the clavicle). These are the supraclavicular lymph nodes.

Oncologists' beliefs about radiotherapy to the supraclavicular nodes have varied over time. Up to the 1990s it was usual for these glands to be treated along with the lymph nodes in the axilla. But then the practice began to fall out of favour. This was partly because of concern about causing more side effects but also from a belief that if the cancer had spread to these glands then it was no longer curable with a local treatment, such as surgery or radiotherapy, and drug treatment offered the only hope of controlling the disease. More recently, however, clinical trials have shown that a cure is still often possible with surgery or radiotherapy (or a combination of the two) if breast cancer has spread to the supraclavicular lymph glands.

This means that if there might be microscopic traces of cancer in the supraclavicular lymph nodes then irradiating them is worth-while and might lead to a cure. The problem is that these microscopic traces are invisible and there is no way of knowing for certain whether they are there or not. Studies have shown that the greater the number of axillary lymph nodes that are found to contain cancer cells the greater the risk of spread to the supraclavicular nodes. This has led to some guidelines suggesting that if four or more lymph nodes under the arm are found to be invaded by cancer cells then radiotherapy to the supraclavicular nodes would be a wise precaution. As is so often the case in breast cancer, there are no fixed rules and no absolute agreement and some other guidelines recommend that if the primary breast cancer is large (more than 5 cm across) or a grade III cancer then radiotherapy to the supraclavicular glands should be given even if only one to three axillary nodes contains cancer cells.

What if I do nothing?

If you have had a breast-sparing operation then there is still a chance that your cancer could come back in the remaining breast tissue. Having radiotherapy greatly reduces this risk but is not a guarantee that the cancer will not come back. If the cancer comes back, whether or not you have had radiotherapy, you will usually be able to have a mastectomy, which still offers a good chance of cure. So not having radiotherapy does not reduce your chance of cure but does increase the risk that at some time in the future you will need a mastectomy and have to lose what remains of your breast. Most women prefer to go for the reassurance and increased security of having radiotherapy but the choice is yours.

After a mastectomy most women will not need radiotherapy, but if it is recommended this will be because your oncologists feel there is a high risk of your cancer coming back in the skin on the front of your chest. If you don't have radiotherapy, and the cancer does come back then usually it can be treated with further surgery followed by radiotherapy without reducing your chance of a long-term cure. Once again the choice is yours but most women opt for the reassurance of having the radiotherapy sooner rather than later.

If radiotherapy to either your axillary or supraclavicular lymph nodes is recommended this will be because there is a risk that they contain microscopic traces of cancer that could spread to other parts of your body. If that happens then a cure becomes more difficult and less certain, so you would be taking quite a risk if you decided not to have this treatment.

6

Drug treatment: who needs it?

The reason for giving drugs after surgery and radiotherapy have dealt with your primary breast cancer is to destroy any microscopic traces of the cancer that might have spread to other parts of your body. But because those minute clusters of cancer cells are completely invisible, there is no way of knowing whether they are there or not. There is no medical test that will tell you and your doctors if your cancer has spread and if you need further treatment. One answer to this problem would be to give drug treatment to all women with early breast cancer. But that treatment, which might be cytotoxic drugs (chemotherapy), hormone treatment or one of the newer targeted therapies or a combination of these different agents, can sometimes go on for years and often involves unpleasant side effects, which occasionally can be severe or even life-threatening. Because of this, oncologists only want to give drug treatment to those women who really need it, those women who do have invisible but potentially lethal spread of their breast cancer. So how can doctors tell who needs treatment if the secondary cancers that they want to treat are undetectable?

The simple answer is that they can't be certain. But what they can do is use information about your primary breast cancer to predict the risk of it already having spread. Back in the 1970s, when drug treatment was first used for early breast cancer, oncologists realized that if the cancer was in one or more of the axillary lymph nodes then the chance of spread to other parts of the body was greater than if those lymph nodes were clear of any cancer cells. So they used the simple rule that if any of the lymph nodes under the arm showed signs of cancer then drug treatment should be given, but if the glands were normal it was not needed.

Over time, research has shown that other factors also alter the risk of distant spread of the disease and that just looking at the axillary lymph nodes is not the answer. We now know that your age, the size of the primary cancer, the grade of the primary cancer and whether or not there are oestrogen or HER2 receptors all alter the chances of the cancer having spread and the lymph nodes under the arm being affected.

With so many different factors affecting the likelihood of your cancer having spread, how do oncologists weigh up the risks and decide whether or not to recommend some type of drug treatment? There are no fixed rules about this and different doctors will do things differently. Some will rely on years of experience and use their judgement. But there are well-established systems they can use to help in their decision-making and we will spend the rest of this chapter looking at these.

The Nottingham Prognostic Index

The Nottingham Prognostic Index (NPI) was first worked out in the early 1980s by a group of surgeons and statisticians working in Nottingham. Its formula is:

$$NPI = (0.2 \times S) + N + G$$

S is the size of the primary cancer, measured in cm. N is the number of lymph nodes under the arm involved with cancer: if there are no lymph nodes affected the score is 1, if one to three nodes are affected the score is 2 and if more than three nodes are affected then the score is 3. G is the grade of the cancer, so a grade I cancer scores 1, a grade II cancer scores 2 and a grade III cancer scores 3. So if a woman had a grade III primary cancer measuring 3 cm, with two lymph nodes involved, her NPI would be 5.6 whereas if a woman had a grade I primary cancer measuring 2 cm with no lymph nodes affected, her score would be 2.4.

Over the years research has shown that the NPI score can be used to predict a woman's chance of surviving 10 years after her breast cancer is diagnosed. So 9 out of 10 of women who have an NPI score of 2.5 or less will be well with no sign of cancer 10 years later, but if the score is more than 5.4 then only about 5 out of 10 women will be alive and free of cancer in 10 years' time.

Oncologists have used these statistics as a way of predicting whether a woman might have microscopic spread of her cancer, saying that the higher the NPI score the more likely it is that those tiny traces of cancer will be present and the greater the need for some form of adjuvant drug treatment. The problem is that there is no agreement about how actually to use the NPI scores: one oncologist might recommend drug treatment to any woman who has a score of 4 or more, another might say they only advise treatment if the score is 4.5 or more and another might only offer chemotherapy if the score is more than 5.

The NPI also has the disadvantage that it takes no account of the woman's age, whether or not her cancer has oestrogen or HER2 receptors, or the type of treatment she might receive. All these things mean that although the NPI has been widely used over the years as a guide to a woman's chance of cure and whether or not she needs drug treatment, it is still only a fairly crude tool. How it is used and what advice is actually given by oncologists varies very much from doctor to doctor.

Adjuvant Online and PREDICT

The Internet gives access to several tools that offer a completely different way of thinking about who may or may not need drugs as part of their treatment for early breast cancer. The first of these was called Adjuvant Online (AoL). This is an American-based system and although it can be accessed in the UK it is only available to doctors. It uses the past results of treatment for thousands of women in the USA to give an idea of what a woman's chance of surviving breast cancer might be.

To use AoL your oncologist goes online and enters key facts about you and your cancer into the system. These include your age and general health, the size and grade of your primary cancer, whether or not it has ER receptors, whether or not any axillary lymph nodes are affected by cancer and if so how many. AoL will then give a figure for the likelihood of surviving 10 years with surgery and radiotherapy. Your oncologist can then choose from a variety of drug therapies and model what effects these have on your survival figure.

In September 2010 the NHS introduced its own online tool: PREDICT. Unlike AoL this is available to everyone – it isn't

How PREDICT works

Ms White is 60 years old and has had surgery and radiotherapy for a 2 cm, grade I primary cancer that was found by breast screening (she did not know she had a lump). Her cancer had not spread to any of the axillary nodes and it had oestrogen receptors (ER+) but no HER2 receptors (HER2–). Putting all this information into PREDICT, the system tells us that in Ms White's situation 96 women out of 100 would be alive with no sign of breast cancer 5 years later if they had surgery and radiotherapy only, with no drug treatment (a 96 per cent chance of being well and cancer-free). Adding cytotoxic chemotherapy and hormone therapy to her treatment would only increase this number to 97 out of 100; in other words it would make virtually no difference to her chances of a cure. Almost certainly Ms White would feel that given all the inconvenience and risk of side effects involved with drug treatment there would be no point in her having cytotoxic drugs or hormones because they would have such a tiny effect on her chance of a cure.

Things are different if we look at Ms Black, who is also 60 years old. She found a lump in her breast that turned out to be a 3 cm, grade III cancer that had spread to three of her axillary lymph nodes. Her cancer was positive for both oestrogen and HER2 receptors (ER+, HER2+). Here, PREDICT tells us that in this situation only 52 women out of 100 would be alive and free of breast cancer 5 years later (a 52 per cent chance of being well and cancer-free); in 48 out of 100 their cancer would have come back, with distant secondary cancers. Giving cytotoxic chemotherapy would mean an extra 12 women would be well 5 years later (offering a 64 per cent chance of being clear). Hormone therapy would help another 11 women (increasing the chance to 75 per cent) and giving the targeted therapy Herceptin would help another 6 women (boosting the chance to 81 per cent). So for Ms Black, having drug treatment would make a real difference to her chance of beating her cancer and it is very likely that she would want to have drug treatment. The PREDICT result also shows how helpful each type of treatment is and what its benefits are likely to be so that you can see how useful, or not, each particular type of treatment might be for you.

just for doctors – so if you want to you can go online to <www.predict.nhs.uk> and try the system. Once again it uses key facts about you and your cancer and will give figures for your chances of surviving both 5 and 10 years with different types of treatment. AoL has been around for some years and most breast cancer specialists are aware of it, but PREDICT was introduced with virtually no publicity by the NHS and most people do not know it exists. Certainly at my talks for Breast Cancer Care none of the women have heard about it and I think many oncologists are not aware of its existence. It is a well-kept secret.

The idea behind both AoL and PREDICT is that your oncologist can put all your details into the system and then print out the results. They can discuss these results with you and give you a copy of the printout so that you can think about your treatment options and what the benefits of each might or might not be.

Systems like PREDICT and AoL are only guides. They still do not say for sure what will happen if you choose a particular pattern of treatment. So for Ms White (see box opposite), although it is very likely indeed that she will be cured by surgery and radiotherapy alone, there is still a 4 per cent (1 in 25) chance that this won't be the case. For Ms Black also, although having drug treatment greatly increases her chance of cure, even if she does have all the treatment on offer there is still about a 20 per cent (1 in 5 chance) that it won't work and her cancer will come back. But these systems do give you and your doctors a good idea of how useful, or useless, the various treatment options might be in your situation and give a very helpful starting point for discussing whether you might benefit from having a particular type of therapy.

Although AoL has been established for more than a decade and PREDICT is universally available, none of the women I have met in my Breast Cancer Care workshops has heard of them and certainly none has been given a printout from either system by their oncologists in order to have an informed discussion about their treatment. It may be that I met a very unrepresentative group of women but this experience does suggest that many oncologists either do not use one of these tools to help decide on treatment or if they do they do not share that information with their patients.

Talking to your oncologist

For Ms Black and Ms White PREDICT gives quite clear information for them to make their choices about treatment: Ms White almost certainly won't want the worry and stress of extra treatment whereas Ms Black is likely to be grateful for the greatly increased chance of cure that drug therapy will offer her. But suppose we look at another lady, Ms Grey, for whom PREDICT shows that cytotoxic and hormone therapy lifts her chance of being well without breast cancer in 5 years time from 80 per cent to 85 per cent. With surgery and radiotherapy she has a very good chance of success but there is still a 1 in 4 risk that her cancer could come back. Treatment reduces the likelihood that this will happen but does not make a dramatic difference. What should she do? What would you do? Ms Grey might have a very clear idea of what she wants and be able to make a choice but she may be uncertain and want to talk things through with her oncologist and get their advice. What will they say?

It may seem hard to believe but oncologists, like all doctors, are only human and they will vary in their views. At one extreme they may feel that their overriding duty is to give the best chance of a cure and so they will have no hesitation in recommending further treatment with cytotoxic drugs and hormones. At the other extreme they may feel that their responsibility is to balance prospects for cure with the risks of side effects, distress and disruption from additional treatment; they will want to put quality of life at the centre of their thinking and they may be much more reluctant to suggest drug therapy. Others will occupy the middle ground, discussing the benefits from and problems with the different options, answering questions and giving information to help you, and them, reach an agreed solution. At the end of the day the decision is yours not theirs; they can advise you but you have the final say. If you feel most comfortable and find it best to say: 'You're my doctor and you know best, I'll trust you and do what you say' then that's fine, but if you want to take time to think things over and make up your mind that is also entirely all right.

Thinking time

It is a general rule that the sooner a cancer is diagnosed and treated the better. The Department of Health has a target that any woman who has been told by her family doctor (GP) that she might have a breast cancer should be seen in a specialist breast clinic at her local hospital within 2 weeks, so that treatment can start as quickly as possible.

But breast cancers usually grow quite slowly. By the time most women have discovered their breast cancer it will have been there for many months, if not several years, although too small to be obvious. There has also been a lot of research showing that a delay in diagnosing and treating breast cancer of between 3 and 6 months seems to have no effect on the chance of a cure.

So on the one hand it seems there is a need for great urgency in finding and treating breast cancer and on the other no need at all to rush things. How can we make sense of this apparent conflict? The answer lies in the old saying, a favourite of my grandmother's, 'make haste slowly'. The various clinic appointments and tests needed to determine whether or not you have a breast cancer, and if so how it needs to be treated, should be done without delay. But they should not be rushed. There is time to do things properly and no need to cut corners in order to save a few days here or there. Getting things right is more important than getting them done in the shortest possible time.

This means there is also time for you to find out about and think about your treatment. You don't need to take instant decisions in the very stressful environment of the hospital clinic, where there is often the feeling of there not being enough time to think straight or fully understand what you are being told. Take a few days to:

- consider what your doctors and nurses have said to you;
- read through the information you have been given;
- talk things through with friends and family;
- possibly explore on the Internet or telephone helplines;
- either decide what to do or make a list of the questions you still need to ask before you can make a decision.

This is far better than giving an instant yes or no in the clinic when your mind is likely to be in a whirl of uncertainty and anxiety.

Taking a few days or even a week or two to get all the facts you need to make up your mind and reach a choice that you are comfortable with and feel is right for you will not reduce your chance of a cure, will not put your life at risk. But it will give you the chance to regain some control at a time when things usually feel completely chaotic, and to plan a course of action that you feel is right for you and is what you want. Your doctors are there to give you advice; it is up to you how you use that advice and what you do with it, and you need time to think to make these decisions. Taking that time is not going to do you any harm.

Second opinion

One day in my clinic in Wolverhampton I was asked by a local GP to see a woman who had just had surgery for her breast cancer and was very anxious to talk about further treatment. I spent the best part of 2 hours going over all the different possibilities with her and her son. At the end of our discussion she thanked me profusely and said, 'I'm so grateful to you Dr Priestman, now I know exactly what to ask Professor X when I see him for my second opinion tomorrow.' I remember I felt a bit irritated that after I had spent so long explaining everything in great detail she still needed another doctor's view of her situation and what she should do. But this was wrong. Everyone has the right to ask for a second opinion.

Most women will feel that with the information they have been given, and after talking things through with their oncologist, possibly their specialist breast care nurse, their family and friends, they are able to make a decision that they are comfortable with. But some will still feel they need another expert's view of things. They may feel unhappy with the advice they have been given, they may just feel confused and want some clarification, or they may need the reassurance of someone else telling them that what they have already been told is right.

If you have anxieties and uncertainties and feel it would help if you could talk to another breast cancer specialist then you can ask

A look into the future

In every normal cell and every cancer cell there is a nucleus. In the nucleus are the chromosomes. On the chromosomes, strung out like pearls on a necklace, are the genes. The genes control the cell and determine how it behaves. In cancer cells the genes have become damaged, or mutated, and this is why cancer cells behave differently from normal cells. The pattern of which genes have been damaged and how they have mutated is different in different cancers. In breast cancer lots of different patterns of gene mutation are possible.

In recent years scientists have learnt how to look at breast cancer cells that have the faulty genes but this is still a very specialized and expensive test only available at a few research centres. But it does offer a hope for the future that doctors and scientists are working on. The idea is to collect information about how breast cancers with different patterns of gene mutation behave: how rapidly they grow, how likely they are to spread and which treatments they respond to. The plan is then to make a databank of this information so that when a woman finds she has a breast cancer it can be tested to work out its pattern of gene mutation. This pattern can then be compared with similar cancers in the databank and this will tell doctors how that cancer is likely to behave, what the best treatment for it will be and what are the chances of success with that treatment.

This is something for the future but the first reports of the use of the research, which is called gene array assay, have begun to appear in the medical journals and there is a good chance that in 5–10 years from now it will become part of the routine care of women with breast cancer. This will mean that any new cancer can be tested to find its pattern of gene mutation, and the hope is that this will give much more accurate information about treatments and their outcomes for individual women with breast cancer than is possible at the moment.

your GP to arrange this. You don't have to go privately or pay: it is a service that is freely available on the NHS. It will mean a further delay and it will usually involve some travelling as most second opinions are with experts at other hospitals. But if you feel that you need another view on things to make an informed choice then these are likely to be minor considerations.

The chances are that you will feel that your medical team have given you all the information and advice you need to make up your mind, and this will be the case for most women. But if you do feel you need the input of another independent expert then asking for a second opinion is an option that is open to you.

7

Chemotherapy: cytotoxic drugs

The use of cytotoxic drugs as part of the treatment of early breast cancer has done more than anything else to boost the chance of a cure over the last 30 years. In 1970 if a woman was told she had early breast cancer then she only had a 50 per cent chance of surviving 5 years. Now that figure is approaching 90 per cent and still rising. Along with the use of hormonal treatments, cytotoxic drugs have been the main reason for this huge improvement in the outlook of women with this disease.

But unfortunately we rarely get something for nothing and the downside of cytotoxic drugs is their side effects. These vary from drug to drug and person to person. One woman may go through a whole course of treatment with virtually no upset at all whereas another woman having exactly the same drugs at exactly the same dose will have severe, possibly even life-threatening problems.

Deciding whether or not to have cytotoxic treatment is a careful balancing act: weighing up the benefits (how much will the drugs increase your chance of being cured) against the risks (the side effects you might experience). In this chapter we will look at how cytotoxic treatment has changed over time, what the possible side effects of treatment may be and some thoughts on how you might make a decision about treatment.

These days there are a lot of different drugs used in the treatment of early breast cancer and it is not possible in a book of this length to give details of them all. Macmillan Cancer Support and Breast Cancer Care have free factsheets, which are also available online, giving comprehensive information on all the drugs mentioned here. Their addresses are given at the end of this book under 'Useful addresses'.

The development of cytotoxic chemotherapy in early breast cancer

Throughout the 1980s and most of the 1990s the most widely used cytotoxic treatment in early breast cancer was a combination of three drugs: cyclophosphamide, methotrexate and fluorouracil. Oncologists shortened these names to CMF. Although the drugs in CMF treatment were always the same there were a lot of variations in the way they were given. Usually all three drugs were given through a drip into a vein over a few minutes on a single day (day 1) and the treatment was then repeated 3 weeks later (day 21). This was repeated six times in all, meaning that the course of treatment lasted about 4 months. But some oncologists gave the cyclophosphamide as a tablet rather than an injection, prescribing either a 7- or 14-day course and increasing the interval between the infusions of methotrexate and fluorouracil to 4 weeks, extending the overall treatment time to about 6 months. And there were lots of other minor differences in the dose and scheduling of the three drugs used by different oncologists.

In the late 1990s clinical trials showed that adding one of two drugs called anthracyclines into the mix could offer a small but definite further increase in the chance of a cure. These two drugs were epirubicin (Pharmorubicin) and doxorubicin (Adriamycin). This development led to the introduction of a number of new recipes for treatment with different drug ingredients. These included FEC (fluorouracil, epirubicin and cyclophosphamide through a drip into a vein once every 3 or 4 weeks for six courses), Epi-CMF (epirubicin intravenously on its own for four doses, once every 3 weeks, followed by CMF intravenously for four doses once every 3 or 4 weeks) and AC (Adriamycin and cyclophosphamide intravenously once every 3 or 4 weeks for four courses).

There was no clear evidence from clinical trials that any one of these or any other combination of the drugs was better than the others, so different oncologists tended to use different schedules depending on their personal experience of what they felt worked best and caused fewest side effects. This meant that women with very similar cancers having treatment at different hospitals could find they were having very different cytotoxic treatments. This was not a case of one getting better treatment than the other and neither, importantly, was it a matter of cost – of one hospital trying to give treatment on the cheap. It was simply a reflection of the fact that there was a range of different treatments to choose from, all of which appeared to be equally good at boosting the chance of cure.

Cytotoxic drug dosing

In the early years of cytotoxic chemotherapy, back in the 1960s, doctors realized there was often only a small difference between the dose that was needed to kill the cancer cells and the dose that caused severe side effects. There was only a slim margin of error: give too large a dose and you might cause life-threatening problems, give too small a dose and the drug would be ineffective against the cancer. So there was a need to tailor the amount of drug given on an individual basis rather than adopt a 'one size fits all' approach.

Research showed that the best way to do this was to adjust the dose according to the person's size and that the best measure of size was the surface area of the body. When thinking about our size, height and weight are the first two things that usually come to mind and body surface area is something that is seldom mentioned. But in working out cytotoxic drug doses (and Herceptin doses) it is extremely important. If you are going to have these drugs your medical team will measure your height and weight and these can then be used to find your surface area, which is measured in square metres. They will then use this to calculate the dose of the drug that is exactly right for you.

This precise way of working out drug doses for cytotoxic drugs and Herceptin doesn't apply to hormone treatments, where the 'one size fits all' approach applies. So, for example, everyone who has the hormone drug tamoxifen will be prescribed 20 milligrams a day of the drug regardless of their height, weight or body surface area.

In recent years the picture has been further complicated by the use of another group of cytotoxic drugs called taxanes. The two drugs that have been given in early breast cancer are docetaxel (Taxotere) and paclitaxel (Taxol). Clinical trials have shown that when either of these drugs is added to the mix there is a further slight increase in the chance of cure. But those studies also show that there is an increased risk of side effects. Having two more drugs available multiplies the possibilities for drug combinations and schedules of treatment but one of the most widely used recipes has been to give AC intravenously for four courses once every 3 weeks followed by docetaxel given intravenously once every 3 weeks for four courses. This is just one example of the many different options for using these drugs and there is no clear evidence for one combination or schedule being the best.

Working out exactly who may benefit from having a taxane added to their treatment is still work in progress. At first it was thought that women whose cancer had oestrogen receptors (ER+) or were aged over 50 years might not get any advantage, but research has shown that this is not true. However, there is still some uncertainty whether women with certain types of breast cancer do or do not have their chance of a cure improved by taxane therapy, and this is still an active area of research.

Downsides

If cytotoxic chemotherapy could be given with a guarantee that there would be no problems and no disruption of day-to-day living then the chances are you would opt to have the treatment even if it only offered a very small chance of making a cure more likely. Unfortunately this isn't the case – cytotoxic drugs do cause side effects and even if those side effects are very minor, just having the treatment involves a considerable amount of inconvenience. You will therefore have to weigh up these negatives against the positive of a reduced risk of your cancer coming back when you make the decision whether or not to have treatment.

Giving a detailed description of all the possible side effects of all the cytotoxic drugs that might be used to treat early breast cancer is beyond the scope of this book but those details are readily available from the charities Macmillan Cancer Support, Breast Cancer Care and Cancer Research UK (see 'Useful addresses'). What we will do here is look at three of the most common and most important side effects of these drugs and the disruption to daily life that treatment often involves. If you ask most people what would be the most upsetting side effects they might get from cytotoxic chemotherapy they are likely to say hair loss and sickness, but doctors would put another problem top of the list: neutropenic sepsis.

Hair loss

Most side effects from cytotoxic drugs vary a lot from person to person, but with hair loss (alopecia) the risk depends entirely on which drugs are given. Some, for example fluorouracil, very seldom cause any hair loss; others, like cyclophosphamide, may cause some thinning of the hair but only lead to very obvious alopecia when higher doses are given; and others, like epirubicin and doxorubicin, almost always cause complete hair loss. One or other of these last two drugs almost always forms part of the cocktail of cytotoxic drugs used to treat early breast cancer, which means that virtually all women who opt for chemotherapy will face this challenge. There are two important things to say here. First, once chemotherapy is over your hair always grows back. This will take some months and very often you hair will look and feel different – a pepper and salt colouring with a wavy or slightly curly look and thicker texture or feel is most common. Second, there are things that can be done to reduce the risk of losing your hair.

Hair loss does not happen instantly. If you are having either epirubicin or doxorubicin then the typical pattern is that you will start to lose your hair about 2–3 weeks after the first dose of the drug. But once that hair loss starts it can be very rapid and you may find that you lose all your hair in a matter of a few days. This will often mean not only losing the hair on your head but also your eyebrows and hair on other parts of your body. The best way to stop this happening is to use something called scalp cooling. There are a number of different ways of doing this but they all involve the same idea of using some type of very cold cap or hat that you wear while having your chemotherapy. These will chill your scalp and reduce the blood supply to the hair follicles so that less of the drug gets to them and the risk of hair loss is reduced. Typically, you would start wearing the cold cap about 30 minutes before your dose of chemotherapy is given and keep it on until somewhere between 30 minutes to 2 hours after the infusion of the drugs is finished – anywhere from around 1 to 3 hours overall. Wearing a cold cap each time you have your chemotherapy doesn't guarantee you won't lose any hair; it works for about half to two-thirds of the women who use it. The rest will lose either some or all of their hair.

Scalp cooling only reduces the risk of losing the hair on your head and does not affect hair loss on other parts of your body. There is no way of knowing in advance who will or will not benefit from wearing these chilled hats but what can be said is that if you don't, then with most cytotoxic treatments in early breast cancer, you will lose your hair. Another point is that some women find the scalp cooling difficult to cope with. The hats themselves can sometimes feel quite uncomfortable and the extreme chilling of the scalp is something that can be unpleasant and may cause headaches, so some women decide they would prefer to lose their hair rather than use the cold cap. If you do lose your hair then it is possible to get wigs supplied by the NHS to disguise your hair loss. Other women prefer to use head scarves, bandannas or hats, and others choose simply to leave their heads uncovered. Both Macmillan Cancer Support and Breast Cancer Care have very helpful booklets and advice on coping with hair loss.

Nausea and vomiting

Feeling sick (nausea) or actually throwing up (vomiting) after cytotoxic treatment is another major worry for women who are thinking about having this as part of the package of care for their breast cancer. Sickness is one is those side effects that is very variable from person to person: if two different women are given exactly the same drugs at exactly the same doses, one might have no upset at all and the other might feel horribly queasy for several days after each treatment.

Happily these days there are extremely good treatments for preventing sickness and these will routinely be given to anyone who is having treatment. These anti-sickness drugs will stop any vomiting for the great majority of women. They are slightly less good at taking away any feelings of nausea but this will usually be very considerably reduced so that it isn't very troublesome. Very occasionally, the routine anti-sickness drugs are not completely effective, but it is usually possible to adjust the dose or change the drug so that the problem can be overcome. There were huge improvements in the drugs available to prevent chemotherapy-induced sickness during the 1990s and things have continued to get better since then. Before that time controlling nausea and vomiting after chemotherapy was a big problem and it is memories of those bad old days that tend to colour a lot of people's thinking. Today, sickness with chemotherapy is a largely preventable side effect.

Neutropenic sepsis

Losing your hair and feeling sick are not fun, but from a medical point of view a far more serious side effect of cytotoxic treatment is neutropenic sepsis – far more serious because it can be life-threatening. Almost all cytotoxic drugs will cause a fall in the number of white cells in the blood: the neutrophils and lymphocytes. This drop in the number of white cells usually happens about 7–10 days after having the drug, and the blood count will be back to normal a couple of weeks later.

Most of the time this is not a problem but occasionally the drug or drugs will cause a really big fall in the white blood cell level. This is important because those white blood cells are our body's main defence against infection, and having too few of them means that infections can develop. Because of the lowered resistance, these infections can rapidly become serious – in a matter of just a few hours. This combination of an infection and a low white cell count is called febrile neutropenia, and if the infection becomes severe it is known as neutropenic sepsis. If someone who is having chemotherapy develops a temperature, feels hot and feverish, and starts to feel unwell, they should always contact their chemotherapy team right away to check they are not developing febrile neutropenia (everyone having chemotherapy will always be given a phone number they can call 24 hours a day if they are worried).

This is very important because if febrile neutropenia is diagnosed and treated quickly (treatment usually means a short stay in hospital with intensive antibiotic therapy), it can easily be controlled. But if there are delays things can get worse very quickly and neutropenic sepsis may develop, which is much harder to treat and can occasionally be fatal. The risk of infection following cytotoxic therapy is far and away the most important and potentially dangerous side effect of the drugs and is something everyone thinking about chemotherapy should be made aware of.

Hospital visits

As well as the chance of having side effects, cytotoxic chemotherapy does involve extra hospital visits that disrupt the day-to-day pattern of life. A typical course of chemotherapy will involve six cycles of the drugs given every 3–4 weeks, so four or five treatments in all. Each cycle will usually mean a visit to hospital for a check-up and a blood test, which will probably take about half the day, and then a visit for the treatment itself. This is normally done as a 'day case' in the chemotherapy unit, which means you will spend most of the day at the hospital. As well as these trips there may be visits in between courses if you have any problems or side effects.

Although this does mean a lot more time at hospital, one benefit many women find is that the nurses who run the chemotherapy units are very supportive and helpful and can often be a great source of strength and reassurance at a very difficult time. There is also the chance to meet other people having treatment, share experiences and problems (and how to cope with them) and make new friends. So for many women the trips to have their chemotherapy are a mixed blessing – the treatment is never really pleasant but going to the unit holds the prospect of meeting a friendly and encouraging group of people who can offer a lot of advice, warmth and comfort.

Making your choice

A few years ago a study in the USA looked at how a group of men made decisions about the treatment they wanted for their prostate cancer. The choice was between surgery to remove their prostate gland (a prostatectomy) or a course of high-dose radiotherapy. The chance of cure was the same with both treatments but both carried the risk of unpleasant side effects. The men had talks with surgeons and oncologists, during which the pros and cons of each treatment were explained and lots of written information about the risks and benefits was given.

Later, they were interviewed to find out what had influenced their final choice of treatment. To the surprise of the researchers most of the men based their decisions on personal experience or the advice of family and friends rather than the expert advice they had been given. They said things like: 'Someone told me radio-therapy can burn you so I'm going to have surgery' or 'I'm terrified of the knife so I choose the radiation' or 'My father had an oper-ation for bowel cancer that cured him so I wanted the surgery' or 'My uncle had radiotherapy for his throat cancer and he was fine so that's why I had it too.'

This is a bit discouraging for those of us who spend a lot of our time offering expert evidence-based information to people with cancer. But what it does show is that we are all individuals, people in our own right who will make up our minds in our own way. This is really important because at the end of the day we have to be comfortable with the decisions we make. We will have to live with the outcomes of those decisions, which may affect us for the rest of our lives, and so it is essential that we are happy about our choices and don't feel we have been pressurized to make choices we did not want to make.

It also means that there isn't a right or wrong choice. We don't all go to the same place for our holidays, we don't all want to watch the same things on television and we don't all eat the same things for Sunday lunch. We are all different and we lead our lives in dif-ferent ways. Who we are determines what we want and what we will do, and no two people are the same.

When it comes to making a choice about whether or not to have cytotoxic chemotherapy you will get lots of expert advice. You will get guidance from your oncologist and your specialist nurse. This will be backed up by written information that you can take home and think about. But only you can make the decision. Sometimes this might be quite easy if figures from PREDICT or AoL (see page 61) suggest that the treatment will greatly increase your chance of cure, or if the figures suggest that treatment will make little or no difference. But even then each of us will set our own limits as to what is a worthwhile difference: for some women, raising their chance of cure from 60 per cent to 65 per cent would make all the inconvenience and risks of chemotherapy acceptable whereas for others it would not.

Figures, numbers and statistics are a help but they do not tell you what to do. Recently, my GP told me that statistics show I have a 20 per cent (1 in 5) chance of a heart attack or stroke in the next

10 years and she suggested that I start taking drugs called statins to reduce this risk. I found it really hard to work out what that 1 in 5 chance really meant for me personally and whether it was a risk that did or did not worry me. I gave it a lot of thought, I looked up some of the research and I talked it through with my wife. In the end I decided to take my chance and not have the statins. Ten years from now I will know if that was right or wrong but I have made the decision and it was my decision.

One other thing to remember in making up your mind is that you can always change your mind later. If you do decide to have the treatment and you find that after one or two courses of the drugs you are getting really nasty side effects or that the whole hassle of extra blood tests and hospital visits is too much to cope with then you can just say no and stop there. It is entirely up to you and what you want.

These last few paragraphs may have been a disappointment if you were expecting that they would tell you whether or not you should have cytotoxic chemotherapy. But the whole point of this section has been to underline the fact that the choice is yours. Get as much or as little expert advice as you feel you need; talk to as many or as few friends and relatives who you feel might help; toss a coin or draw a lot, but in the end make the decision that feels right for you and that you are comfortable with. There isn't a right or wrong choice – there is only your choice.

8

Hormone therapy

The use of hormone therapy in early breast cancer has gone hand in hand with cytotoxic therapy to boost the chance of cure and over the last 40 years has made a huge contribution to the improvement in outcomes for people with the disease. However, hormone therapy only works if the breast cancer has oestrogen receptors – if it is ER+. If the cancer doesn't have oestrogen receptors, if it is ER–, then the treatment will not work. Luckily most breast cancers are ER+, but for about 1 in 4 women with breast cancer who have ER– tumours the treatment will not help. These days all breast cancers are tested when they are first discovered to see if they are ER+ or ER–, so you will know immediately if hormone treatment might be for you.

Like all drugs the hormone therapies do have side effects, and once again it is a matter of weighing up the advantages and disadvantages of treatment in order to decide whether or not to go ahead.

The development of hormone therapy in early breast cancer

Like cytotoxic chemotherapy, hormone therapy first began to be used to treat early breast cancer in the late 1970s. At that time the choice of treatments was simple: if a woman was still seeing her periods (if she was premenopausal) then she would be offered an oophorectomy, an operation to take away her ovaries and bring on the menopause (sometimes radiotherapy to the ovaries was used as an alternative: a radiation menopause). If a woman was past the menopause (if she was postmenopausal) then the treatment was the drug tamoxifen, given as a tablet once a day. Having your ovaries removed or irradiated was something that could not be reversed, the change was permanent, but with tamoxifen there was uncertainty over how long it should be given. At first it was prescribed for 2 years but then clinical trials suggested it was more effective if it was given for 5 years, and this became the norm.

Since that time things have become more complicated. These days, oophorectomy and radiation menopauses have been largely replaced by the drug goserelin (Zoladex), which acts on the pituitary gland to bring on a 'chemical menopause' and stop the ovaries working. Unlike surgery and radiotherapy the effects of Zoladex are reversible, so if it is stopped the periods will start again a few months later. We also know now that tamoxifen also works in younger women and will block the effects of oestrogen even if

Cytotoxic chemotherapy or hormone therapy for younger women?

If you are a younger woman still seeing your periods, in other words if you are premenopausal, and you need drug treatment to reduce the risk of your breast cancer coming back, is it better to have cytotoxic chemotherapy or hormone therapy? Over the years lots of clinical trials have been done to try and answer this question. Overall the results seem to show that chemotherapy and hormone therapy are equally good at improving your chances of a cure. Despite these statistics most oncologists recommend cytotoxic chemotherapy rather than hormones (though sometimes a combination of the two may be suggested).

Why this is the case is difficult to explain. Some oncologists just believe the chemotherapy is better even though there is no proof. A slightly more scientific argument is that clinical trials take many years to complete. This means that even the most recent results are from trials using older combinations of cytotoxic drugs and it could be argued that using more up-to-date treatments would give better outcomes and show a greater benefit than hormone therapy. The answer is that nobody knows for sure. For this reason the current NICE guidance of giving tamoxifen and cytotoxic chemotherapy seems like good advice, but if you absolutely cannot face the thought of chemotherapy then having hormone therapy to stop you producing oestrogen is still a very good alternative and there really is no strong evidence that it is any less effective.

they are still seeing their periods. And then we have the aromatase inhibitor group of drugs (anastrozole – Arimidex, exemestane – Aromasin and letrozole – Femara), which stop oestrogen production in women who are past the menopause and so offer an alternative to tamoxifen for this age group.

How these different drugs are used at the present time is quite complicated and there is quite a lot of debate and controversy about what is best. Perhaps the easiest way to talk about this is to describe the current guidance from the National Institute for Health and Clinical Excellence (NICE). The NICE guidance says that premenopausal women having cytotoxic chemotherapy should receive tamoxifen for 5 years after their chemotherapy. If they have decided not to have cytotoxic chemotherapy then they should have Zoladex and tamoxifen for 5 years. Women who are past their menopause and who have a moderate to high risk of their cancer coming back should have Arimidex, Aromasin or Femara for 5 years. If there is a medical reason why they should not have one of these drugs then tamoxifen can be used as an alternative. Women who are postmenopausal and have a low risk of their cancer coming back probably don't need hormone therapy.

NICE also says that for those women who have DCIS, the early non-invasive form of breast cancer, there is no need for hormone therapy and it should not be given.

The NICE guidance is helpful but it is only guidance, not a set of rules, and it does leave some questions unanswered. For example, it does not spell out what a 'low risk' or 'high risk' of cancer coming back actually means. Another thing that is uncertain is the use of what has become known as sequential therapy. Sequential therapy means giving tamoxifen for 2–5 years and then following this with one of the aromatase inhibitors for a further 3–5 years. Some clinical trials have suggested that this may be slightly more effective than giving either tamoxifen or an aromatase inhibitor on their own for 5 years. But whether it really is better and who might benefit from it is uncertain at the present time.

With so many different options in terms of both drugs and timing of treatment, let me try and summarize the picture, always remembering that everyone's treatment is worked out just for them and there will always be variations from person to person.

Tamoxifen or an aromatase inhibitor?

It would be nice to believe that experts know what is best and always agree. Unfortunately, in many aspects of early breast cancer and its treatment this isn't true. Nowhere is this more so than in the question of whether aromatase inhibitors (Arimidex, Aromasin or Femara) are better than tamoxifen for stopping the cancer coming back. Despite masses of facts and figures from any number of clinical trials, leading authorities disagree on the answer.

One of the problems is that none of these clinical trials has been running long enough to show that more women are cured with one drug or the other. Because of this a different way has been used to measure success – whether or not the cancer has come back during the first 2 or 3 years of treatment. The statistics show a small benefit for the aromatase inhibitors: roughly speaking, if 100 women take either tamoxifen or an aromatase inhibitor then about 10 of those taking tamoxifen will find their cancer has come back within 3 years whereas only about 8 of those on an aromatase inhibitor will have a relapse. This is a small difference but because the trials include large numbers of women the results are 'statistically significant', which might suggest that there is no contest between the two therapies and aromatase inhibitors are better.

But these figures only tell us about cancer coming back and not about cure. And they only tell us about the first 2 or 3 years after treatment, and things may change over a longer time. For example, it is possible that if the women in the trials were studied at 10 years rather than 2 or 3 years, tamoxifen might prove to be more effective. This is where understanding breast cancer research gets confusing but the important thing is that it should not be worrying. Tamoxifen and the aromatase inhibitors are very effective treatments for curing breast cancer. The fact that there is so much uncertainty over which is better shows that there is very little to choose between them and either type of drug has an excellent chance of success.

Because there is so little difference in the effectiveness of tamoxifen and aromatase inhibitors, one thing that can help in deciding which to have is their side effects; these are discussed on pages 83–6.

- If you are still seeing your periods and your doctors think you need drug treatment to reduce the risk of your cancer coming back, they are likely to recommend cytotoxic chemotherapy. If they think you would also benefit from hormone treatment they will probably suggest adding tamoxifen for 5 years. If, for whatever reason, you decide you do not want the cytotoxic drugs then they will recommend tamoxifen plus Zoladex for 5 years.
- If you are a postmenopausal woman and you need drug treatment to reduce the risk of your cancer coming back, this may be either cytotoxic chemotherapy followed by hormone treatment, or hormone treatment on its own. In either case your doctors will probably suggest an aromatase inhibitor as the first choice for a 5-year period. But other options are tamoxifen for 5 years or tamoxifen for 2 or 3 years followed by an aromatase inhibitor for 3–5 years.

Although experts disagree on many things in the treatment of breast cancer, everyone believes that hormone therapy should be given for at least 5 years. But there is good evidence that things are different in the real world. In recent years a number of studies have been published from various countries, all of which show the same thing: after 2 years about half the women who have been prescribed hormonal drugs have stopped taking them. They often don't tell their doctors but the truth is they don't renew their prescriptions and simply opt out of treatment. There are likely to be lots of different reasons for this but almost certainly one of the main ones is the side effects of the drugs.

Downsides

Menopausal symptoms

When tamoxifen first appeared in the early 1970s it was hailed as the wonder drug for breast cancer. This was partly because it was a very effective therapy but also because it had almost no side effects. But as time went on it was realized that this was not entirely true and it could cause some quite serious problems, which we will look at later in this section.

But these problems were uncommon and the feeling was that for most women the drug was extremely safe. Safe, maybe, but not without problems. From the outset many women taking tamoxifen complained about menopausal symptoms – they developed frequent and often severe hot flushes, vaginal dryness, loss of sex drive, mood swings, memory problems, loss of concentration and just felt generally wretched. In the male-dominated world of breast cancer medicine at the time, these were largely dismissed as 'women's problems' and not taken seriously as side effects. Happily, over time attitudes have changed, but not everywhere, and probably not enough. Many doctors still underrate the distress that these menopausal symptoms can cause and that for some women they can make life an absolute misery and even, on occasions, lead to thoughts of suicide.

Not all women will get these menopausal symptoms from tamoxifen but a substantial minority do, and although they are less common with the aromatase inhibitors (Arimidex, Aromasin and Femara), they do still often occur. For younger women who are having Zoladex injections these will also bring on menopausal symptoms which, once again, are often more severe than with a natural menopause.

If you do get menopausal symptoms there is a lot that can be done to try and help. This includes changing to a different brand or taking the drug at a different time of day if you are on tamoxifen, or changing to a different drug (from tamoxifen to an aromatase inhibitor or vice versa). There are also various drugs that can be given to try and counteract the hot flushes and other problems. Sometimes these interventions work but sometimes they don't and women are left with the unhelpful advice that it is just something they have got to learn to live with. As we have seen in the previous section, many women don't cope and simply give up the treatment.

One of the difficulties is the length of the treatment. Unlike cytotoxic chemotherapy, which goes on for only a few months, these are drugs that you are told you have to take for at least 5 years, and 5 years is a long, long time to suffer the constant upset of feeling continuously menopausal. We'll talk more about this in the next section.

Although these menopausal symptoms are the most common side effect of hormone therapies there are other problems that can occur with the drugs.

Blood clots and womb cancer

Two further problems with tamoxifen are blood clots and womb cancer. Taking tamoxifen does slightly increase the risk of developing blood clots (thrombosis). This can cause local pain, swelling and discomfort, most often in the veins of the legs, and occasionally more serious problems like strokes or a blood clot on the lungs (a pulmonary embolus). For the great majority of women this is not going to happen and it is a very uncommon complication of treatment, but if you have had problems with blood clots or thrombosis in the past this does increase your risk. Nowadays, any woman who is going to have tamoxifen should always be asked about her medical history before the drug is prescribed, to make sure she is not at greater than normal risk of developing blood clots. If there have been any episodes of thrombosis in the past the drug should not be given.

It was only after tamoxifen had been widely used for some years that doctors began to realize it could cause womb cancer. We now know that about 1 in every 500 women who take tamoxifen for more than 2 years are at risk of developing a cancer of their womb (also called uterine or endometrial cancer). For this reason all women who take the drug should be warned that if they see any unusual vaginal bleeding they should let their doctors know at once so that they can be checked to make sure they have not developed a cancer of their uterus. The two good things about this complication of treatment are that it is very uncommon and that if a womb cancer is discovered then having a hysterectomy (an operation to take away the womb) almost always leads to a complete cure.

Bone thinning and muscle and joint pain

The aromatase inhibitors also unfortunately have possible side effects (in addition to the risk of menopausal symptoms). These include bone thinning and muscle and joint pain. When women pass the menopause their ovaries stop working and the level of the female hormone oestrogen in their blood falls dramatically. Taking an aromatase inhibitor lowers the oestrogen level even further. Oestrogen keeps the bones healthy and strong, so when oestrogen levels are low there is an increased risk of bone thinning (osteoporosis) and this in turn leads to an increased risk that bones might break (fracture).

Soon after they were introduced, studies showed that aromatase inhibitors did increase a woman's risk of osteoporosis and fracture, so now any woman who is going to have one of these drugs should have a test called a bone density, or DXA, scan to check their bone health. If their bones are strong and there is no sign of osteoporosis then it is all right to have the drug but if there is evidence of definite osteoporosis and bone thinning then it is best avoided and tamoxifen given instead (tamoxifen does not cause bone thinning and may even help strengthen the bones). Sometimes the scan will show that although there isn't actual osteoporosis the bone is not as healthy as it should be and in this situation doctors will often prescribe calcium supplements and vitamin D to help build up and protect the bone, as well as giving an aromatase inhibitor.

Pain in the muscles and joints, called arthralgia, is a problem that about 1 in 3 women who take an aromatase inhibitor will experience. It usually comes on about 2 months after starting treatment and sometimes it will wear off after a few months but sometimes it doesn't. Often, a mild painkiller like paracetamol or an anti-inflammatory drug like ibuprofen will ease the discomfort but for a few women the problem will be sufficiently troublesome that they will have to stop taking the drug and change to something else, like tamoxifen.

This list of side effects isn't the full story; tamoxifen and the aromatase inhibitors do occasionally cause other problems but these are much less common.

Making your choice

Deciding whether or not to have hormonal therapy is relatively easy; what may be more difficult is deciding whether or not to continue with it once you have started. Let me explain.

Compared with cytotoxic chemotherapy, hormone treatment is relatively easy to cope with, at least at the beginning. It only means taking a tablet once a day if you are having tamoxifen or an aromatase inhibitor, and even if you are having Zoladex this is only an injection once every 3 months. You don't need regular blood tests, and clinic visits will be every few months rather than every few weeks. And side effects, if they occur at all, often develop slowly over weeks or months whereas with cytotoxic treatment you may feel sick and ill within an hour or so of starting the drugs. Actually having the treatment is therefore very straightforward and has little or no effect on day-to-day life. So it is easy to say yes if your oncologist suggests it might be helpful for you.

The problem is what happens if, when you have been taking the treatment for a while, you develop troublesome side effects like menopausal symptoms – hot flushes, night sweats, mood swings, vaginal dryness, loss of interest in sex, difficulty concentrating – or muscle and joint pains or less common upsets like sickness or headaches. If you are having difficulties the first thing to do is to talk to your oncologist or specialist nurse and they will be able to suggest ways to try to help ease the problem.

Most women taking hormone treatment won't have much in the way of side effects and will cope with the drugs without any disruption to everyday life. For those who do develop symptoms the various measures suggested by their medical team will make things sufficiently bearable to carry on without any great inconvenience. But for a small, very important minority, really upsetting symptoms will persist and life will be a misery.

If you are unlucky enough to be in this small group of women then it is very important to talk to your oncologist and ask just how important it is that you are on the treatment. Because hormone drugs are easy to take and often trouble-free, oncologists tend to have a far lower threshold of benefit for recommending them than they do for cytotoxic chemotherapy. Provided that your cancer has oestrogen receptors (is ER+) then you may be offered hormone therapy even if you are at very low risk of your cancer coming back, the thinking being that as it is easy to take and usually well tolerated then even if it only has a tiny benefit you may as well take it. But if you have side effects that are not easily controlled or eased then you need to find out from your oncologist how important it really is that you continue the treatment. They can use systems like Adjuvant Online or PREDICT (see page 61) to give you an idea of how valuable the drugs are to you personally. If the figures suggest your chance of a cure is only slightly improved by taking the hormone treatment then you may well feel that stopping the drugs is perfectly reasonable. For example, if you already have a 95 per cent chance of a cure and taking hormones – probably for 5 years or more, on top of all the problems you are living with – raises that figure to 97 per cent then giving up ought to be a very easy decision. Similarly, if the figures suggest that without hormones you chance of cure is only 30 per cent but with the drugs this is boosted to 90 per cent then gritting your teeth and carrying on for as long as you can bear is likely to be your choice.

What is more difficult is the choice when you are somewhere in between these extremes: if your chance of cure without hormone drugs is 70 per cent and with them it is 80 per cent. What would you do? I am afraid I can't answer that for you: it is your decision. And each of us will balance things differently. Only you know how much the side effects are interfering with your quality of life and how ill you feel with them, and only you know how important it is to squeeze every last drop of benefit from treatment to get every last possible chance of a cure. It's your choice and only you can make it, but the important thing is to make sure you have all the facts and figures and all the information you need from your oncologist for you to make that decision.

A final point to make here is that I often find that women who have been taking hormone therapy for a while and are having a really hard time with side effects still find it very difficult to think about giving up the drugs, even if they are only offering the tiniest increase in their chance of cure. They often say that as their cancer has not come back while they have been on the drugs they are worried that if they stop it will recur, with the double worry that not only would the cancer be back but it would be their fault because they stopped the drugs. The logic of medical statistics, numbers from AoL or PREDICT, or reassurances from your oncologist may or may not help ease these worries and let you make a decision you are comfortable with. There is no right or wrong answer, there is only the choice that you feel is right for you and that you will be able to live with.

9

Targeted therapy

Targeted therapies are newer drugs that first began to appear at the end of the 1990s. They target abnormalities in cancer cells and unlike the cytotoxic drugs have little or no effect on the growth of normal cells. This means that they do not cause so many side effects but unfortunately, like all drugs, they do have some adverse effects for some people.

At the present time only one targeted therapy, trastuzumab (Herceptin), has been approved by NICE in England and Wales for the treatment of breast cancer. Others, like lapatinib (Tyverb) and bevacizumab (Avastin), are being used in clinical trials and many more compounds are waiting in the wings. Whether biological therapies will transform the way breast cancer is treated in the future remains to be seen. For the moment the only evidence we have to go on is for Herceptin, and we will look at this drug in the rest of this chapter.

Herceptin

By the early 2000s Herceptin was being used in the treatment of advanced breast cancer. In 2005 two clinical trials reported the first results of using the drug as an adjuvant treatment, alongside cytotoxic chemotherapy, in women with early breast cancer. These reports attracted worldwide publicity and were blown out of all proportion by the media, giving people the idea that Herceptin was the new miracle cure for breast cancer. This is simply not true. It is a useful drug for a few people but is no magic bullet.

Herceptin only works if the breast cancer cells have HER2 receptors (HER2+ cancers). Only about 1 in 3 to 1 in 4 breast cancers are HER2+. This means that for most women with early breast cancer, Herceptin won't work and is of no value. The latest clinical trial figures suggest that, for those women who do have HER2+

tumours, adding Herceptin to existing drug treatments (cytotoxic and hormone therapies) might increase their chance of a cure by about 4 per cent. In other words for every 100 women who get the drug 4 more will be cured. On the other hand this also means that of every 100 women who have Herceptin, only 4 get any benefit from it and for the other 96 there is just inconvenience and the risk of side effects. What is the inconvenience and what are the side effects?

Downsides

Herceptin is usually given as an infusion (drip) into a vein once every 3 weeks. There is still some uncertainty as to how long it should be given for, and the length of treatment varies from 4 months to 2 years, although most oncologists are giving it for about a year. Herceptin is normally given after your course of cytotoxic chemotherapy has ended and so this means an additional period of hospital visits. The main risk with Herceptin is that it can cause damage to your heart, which can lead to heart failure. Heart failure doesn't mean that your heart stops working; it is not the same as a heart attack. But it does mean that your heart works less efficiently and this can lead to problems, like being short of breath and very tired, and developing a build-up of fluid in the body, which most often shows up as swelling of your ankles. It can be treated with various drugs but is obviously not a good thing to have if you can avoid it.

Studies have shown that overall about 1 in 10 women having Herceptin get some signs of heart damage and for about 1 in 50 this leads to symptoms of heart failure. Although there is still a bit of uncertainty it does look as though all these changes disappear if you stop the drug and there is no long-lasting effect on your heart. A number of things have now been shown to increase the risk of heart problems with Herceptin and these include a history of previous heart disease, having poorly controlled high blood pressure, being over 60 years old and being overweight.

To reduce the risk as far as possible all women who are considered for Herceptin treatment now have special tests to check that their heart is healthy and working well before they are offered the drug.

Once treatment has started, these tests are usually repeated about once every 3 months to make sure there are no early signs of heart damage from Herceptin.

Although heart failure is the most serious side effect of Herceptin it can cause other problems such as allergic reactions at the time of the infusion of the drug, headaches, muscle pains, changes in the way things taste and a range of other upsets, but these are usually not serious or particularly troublesome.

Making your choice

Only women whose breast cancer is HER2+ will have to make this decision so it will not be an issue for most people. If your cancer is HER2+ and the possibility of Herceptin has been suggested then your oncologist will be able to give you more information about how valuable the extra treatment might be. I have already mentioned Adjuvant Online and PREDICT as guides that can be used to give a rough idea of how important, or otherwise, a particular treatment will be. At the time of writing Adjuvant Online still does not include Herceptin among its choice of treatments but the drug is included in PREDICT (which is the system you can go online to look at yourself). For most women the likelihood is that Herceptin will probably be the icing on the cake compared with treatments like cytotoxic therapy and hormone treatment, which will usually be much more important for boosting your chance of a cure. On average, Herceptin is likely to increase the chance of stopping the cancer coming back by about 4 per cent. Another way of looking at this is that there is only about a 25 to 1 chance that it will make a difference for you.

For some women, increasing their chance of cure by just 1 per cent is worthwhile; doing everything possible to reduce the risk of the cancer coming back is all important. For others the inconvenience and the fact that there might be side effects is just too much hassle to make the possibility of a benefit worthwhile. As ever the decision is yours and only you can work out what your priorities are and what matters to you. Having said this, although the improvement in the chance of a cure that Herceptin gives is relatively small, the disruption of having a treatment once every 3 weeks is not too troublesome; the tests that will be done before and during treatment will keep any risk of damage to your heart to an absolute minimum; and if any signs of a problem do appear then if you stop the drug everything should go back to normal very rapidly. In other words although there may not be that much to gain there is also not much to lose by giving the drug a try and if you find, for whatever reason, that you are not really coping then you can always stop the treatment at any time.

10

Complementary and alternative treatments

Surgery, radiotherapy and chemotherapy are the cornerstones of medical treatment for cancer. But many people choose to explore other approaches. These may be either complementary or alternative therapies. Complementary therapies are usually holistic treatments used alongside conventional therapies. They are an addition to the normal cancer treatments and are not used instead of them. There is a wide range of reasons why people turn to these therapies: they may help ease some of the side effects of the cancer and its treatment and they can offer a sense of control – a feeling that you are free to make choices about what you want and how you want to do it at a time when it can feel that doctors, hospitals and your illness are taking over your life. They also often feel good and add to your overall quality of life.

Alternative therapies are different from complementary therapies. Alternative therapies are treatments that people choose instead of the standard treatments. As a medical doctor I find it hard to understand why people want to go down this road. Perhaps if you have very advanced cancer and your doctors have said there is nothing more to be offered by way of active treatment then alternative therapies may offer a straw to clutch at, a hope that something completely different might help. But at the end of the day there is no scientific evidence that any of these treatments work, either as cures for cancer or ways of increasing survival in the terminal stages of the illness. But some people do believe passionately in these alternative therapies.

Complementary therapies

There is a huge range of complementary therapies, far too many to talk about in this short book, but I will highlight a few of the more widely used treatments. These include mind–body therapies, physical therapies and exercise therapies.

Mind–body therapies are organized around the idea of relaxation – putting the mind and body at peace so that the stresses of cancer and its treatment can, for a short time at least, be put to one side, allowing calmer thoughts and sensations to take over. This might be done simply by relaxation classes in a quiet environment with gently reassuring and supportive advice from an expert to put you at ease. Or it might take the form of meditation or use art or music as distractions to take your mind away from thoughts of illness and all its problems. Another line of approach is hypnotherapy. This doesn't mean going into a trance and losing control but is often no more than restful conversation designed to put you at peace and help you overcome anxieties and tensions. Although I have said I cannot approve of alternative therapies, I do think many complementary therapies can be very helpful and certainly in my own experience I found hypnotherapy helped me to overcome my fear of flying.

Physical therapies involve people actually doing things to you. This may be with various types of massage or with acupuncture. There are many different types of massage and they can vary from the very gentle to the quite vigorous, but they can be very soothing and help your muscles relax and release stress and tension from the body. Aromatherapy uses aromatic herbs and flower extracts mixed into oils that can be massaged into the skin or inhaled through a diffuser. Reflexology is another special form of massage based on the belief that the different parts of the body are represented on different parts of the feet and that by rubbing and pressing these different areas you can channel energy through those parts of the body and soothe and heal them. For some years I had regular reflexology sessions to try and help my asthma. If I am honest I have to say I don't think they helped with my breathing problems but they were the most wonderfully restorative experiences after a long day in the clinic and overall I certainly felt better for them. I have also tried acupuncture but did not find this a very pleasant experience. It involves having special needles put into your skin in certain areas along 'energy pathways' that the ancient Chinese believed affected the functioning of our organs. Some people have found that it helps to ease some of the side effects of cancer treatment, like sickness and nausea, so it may be that sometimes the small amount of discomfort involved can be worthwhile.

Exercise therapies may sound rather too energetic but they include activities like yoga, t'ai chi and qigong. The general idea of these is to use changes in posture, gentle (generally) movement and breathing control to put your body and in turn your mind into a less stressed, healthier, state.

Hospitals vary in their attitude to complementary therapies. Some cancer departments offer treatments like aromatherapy, relaxation classes and reflexology to their patients but others have no facilities for any of these therapies. This means you may have to do some local research to find out about therapists and their availability. Your GP or specialist nurse may well be able to point you in the right direction and Macmillan Cancer Support has an excellent free booklet on complementary and alternative therapies, which has more information about the treatments and where to find them (see 'Useful addresses').

Complementary therapies are an add-on; they supplement your core cancer treatment but for many people they offer a lot of benefit. They won't make your surgery, radiotherapy or chemotherapy more effective but they may help you cope with them better, may possibly ease their side effects, will introduce you to new people with different ideas and approaches and can be fun and very enjoyable.

Alternative therapies

If I have sounded enthusiastic about complementary therapies I am going to sound very negative about alternative therapies. There is not a scrap of real evidence that these make any difference to the outcome for people with cancer – they don't make a cure more likely and they don't reduce the chance of cancer coming back. But the lack of scientific proof of their benefit doesn't stop countless different people and organizations making claims for their particular remedies and treatments, and the advent of the Internet has increased the number of these quack treatments and eccentric theories.

It is impossible to list all the different 'treatments' on offer. They include countless medicines very often based on plant extracts like laetrile (from apricot stones), iscador (from mistletoe) and essiac (a mixture including burdock root and rhubarb). They are often backed up by attractive-looking clinics, convincing staff (sometimes medically qualified) and reports and publications that look quite scientific. But no one has ever been able to prove they work.

The same is true of the numerous special diets that make up another range of alternative therapies, along with vitamin and other nutritional supplements. A healthy diet with plenty of fresh fruit and vegetables and relatively small amounts of red meat and alcohol helps keep us fit and reduces the risk of all manner of illnesses, including cancer. But we don't need to go to private clinics or pay large sums of money to be told this.

This last point is worth emphasizing. All these alternative therapies involve payment, they definitely are not available on the NHS and sometimes the amounts demanded are very considerable.

One other thing to mention is that sometimes the alternative remedies can be thoroughly unpleasant – the prospect of, for example, coffee enemas or extreme diets is not instantly appealing. One of the problems here is that once people start a treatment they then worry about giving it up, although they find it upsetting, in case this means their cancer will come back. In this way people can find themselves in a vicious circle where they hate the treatment they are having but are too frightened to stop it.

I have had my say and there will be lots of alternative therapists out there saying that this is just what they would expect a medical doctor to say and that I am just narrow-minded and prejudiced. But anyone who abandons conventional treatment for their cancer may be attracted by holistic alternatives and the mystique that surrounds them but, in my opinion, they will gain no benefit in terms of cancer treatment and may end up with a lot of expense, discomfort and, finally, disappointment.

11

If breast cancer comes back: advanced breast cancer

The good news is that more than 8 out of every 10 women who are diagnosed with breast cancer today will be completely cured. But this does mean that there is a very important minority for whom a cure will not be possible because their cancer is too advanced and has spread beyond the breast and the nearby lymph nodes to other parts of their body.

This group of women with advanced breast cancer is partly made up of those whose tumour had already spread and formed secondary cancers (metastases) in other organs at the time their cancer was first discovered: just under 1 in every 20 women will have advanced breast cancer when their disease is first diagnosed. But by far the largest part of this group are women who have had a breast cancer treated with surgery, and probably radiotherapy and drugs as well, but whose cancer has come back in the form of metastases in other parts of the body.

If breast cancer does come back this is most likely in the early years after treatment. Recurrences of the disease are uncommon after 5 years and rare after 10 years. If a breast cancer does spread to other parts of the body, the most likely place to be affected is the bones, and the bones most likely to be involved are the spine, pelvis, skull, ribs and thigh bones (femurs). Other organs where metastases are common are the liver, lungs and brain.

Usually a number of secondary cancers will develop: it is very uncommon to have just a single solitary metastasis. The exact number of secondaries varies a lot, from just a few tumours to several dozen or more. But many of these will cause little or no trouble. For instance, when breast cancer spreads to the bones, scans and X-rays will usually show a number of metastases in different parts of the skeleton but only one or two of these are likely to give rise to any pain or discomfort and most will remain silent.

These secondary cancers are made up of breast cancer tissue and although they may be in the lung or liver or elsewhere they behave like breast cancer, not like lung or liver cancer. This is something that very often confuses people, including the media. A breast cancer that has spread to the bone is very different in the way it behaves and the treatment it needs from a cancer that started in the bone – a primary bone cancer. In the same way, a secondary breast cancer in the liver, lung or brain is completely different from a primary cancer of any of those organs.

Second breast cancers

Happily these days the great majority of women who develop early breast cancer will be completely cured. But for the unlucky few the cancer may come back. This most often happens when secondary breast cancer develops with new tumours appearing in other parts of the body: metastatic breast cancer. I talk about this in more detail in the rest of this chapter but another, less common way in which breast cancer can come back is when someone develops a new cancer in their other breast.

Statistics show that women who have had a cancer in one breast are more likely to get a cancer in their other breast than the rest of the female population. During each of the first 10 years after a breast cancer has been found, 1 in every 100 women will find a new cancer in her other breast. This means that if you have had a breast cancer diagnosed then in the next decade you have a 10 per cent (1 in 10) chance of finding a second breast cancer.

Experts have debated whether these second breast cancers are tumours that have spread from the primary breast cancer or are completely new growths. Although there is still some uncertainty, most experts believe that if the second cancer appears within 2 years of the first cancer being found then it is part of that initial cancerous process and has spread from the first cancer. If the new cancer is discovered more than 2 years after the first one then the expert view is that this really is a completely new cancer.

Whether it is a spread from the original cancer or a completely new cancer most second breast cancers are found in the 2 years after the first cancer was diagnosed and the risk slowly reduces after this but doesn't disappear until about 20 years later. However, the good news is that as anyone who has had a breast cancer treated will be having careful check-ups, with regular mammograms, second breast cancers are usually discovered when they are still at a very early stage and highly curable. So although having a second breast cancer is upsetting, treatment is effective and all should be well.

What are your treatment options?

The first line of treatment for secondary breast cancer is drug therapy. This is because the treatment needs to be able to spread through the bloodstream to reach all parts of the body, wherever the metastases might be. Very rarely tests might show that there seems to be only a single secondary in a particular organ and on these occasions surgery might be possible to remove it, but this is extremely uncommon.

For those women whose primary (original) breast cancer contained oestrogen receptors (ER+), their secondary cancers will almost certainly also be ER+ and so they are likely to be sensitive to hormone treatment. This means that for those women who had ER+ primary cancers and are past their menopause, one of the aromatase inhibitors (Arimidex, Aromasin or Femara) is likely to be recommended, to be taken as a daily tablet. For women who are still seeing their periods (who are premenopausal) either tamoxifen or Zoladex or a combination of the two hormonal therapies are options.

These drugs will be given for as long as they appear to be controlling the disease, which may be anywhere from a few months to a number of years. When things get out of control, either with new secondaries appearing or worsening symptoms from existing tumours, then swapping from one hormone drug to another is an option if things are changing fairly slowly, which can often bring about a further period of remission and improvement.

For those women whose cancers are not ER+, or for the small number of women with ER+ tumours whose secondaries seem to be growing very rapidly with the possibility of life-threatening problems, then cytotoxic drugs are the best approach. The exact choice of which drugs to use will depend on what treatment has or has not been given in the past, when the initial primary breast cancer was treated, but there is a wide range of drugs and combination of drugs that can be used.

If, as is very often the case, the breast cancer has spread to the bones then most oncologists will recommend starting on the bisphosphonates (see pages 32–3) as well as having hormone therapy or cytotoxic therapy. These drugs are useful because they help strengthen the bones and reduce the risk of possible breaks (fractures), help with controlling bone pain and also help prevent an important complication of bone secondaries called hypercalcaemia. Hypercalcaemia is when large amounts of calcium leak out of the bone into the bloodstream, which can cause upsetting symptoms like feeling sick, vomiting, becoming confused and generally feeling very unwell.

Radiotherapy can sometimes help to ease symptoms. If pain in a particular bone is a problem then a single radiotherapy treatment will often be enough to ease this. A short course of radiotherapy, possibly with only a couple treatments, can often help control any symptoms from secondary cancers in the brain.

As well as these different treatments that directly help control the cancer there will be a range of medications on offer to relieve any upsetting symptoms. Painkillers ranging in strength from paracetamol to morphine may be needed and there are very effective compounds to stop any nausea or vomiting. Steroids, which have such a bad reputation when taken illegally by sportsmen and women, can sometimes be very beneficial: increasing appetite, increasing energy levels and acting as a very effective general tonic.

What if I do nothing?

I am afraid that here you have to face a very bitter truth. Once breast cancer has spread beyond the nearby lymph nodes, in the axilla or above the collarbone, to the bones or other organs then it can no longer be cured. There is no treatment, despite occasional claims made on the Internet for alternative therapies that can get rid of the cancer for all time. This means that unless some other illness or accident intervenes you will eventually die from your breast cancer.

This is devastating news and usually there will be a lot of help and support on offer from your medical team to help you cope with the trauma of this situation. Charities like Macmillan Cancer Support and Breast Cancer Care also offer advice and comfort with booklets and leaflets giving lots of valuable information, and they have helplines where you can talk to a sympathetic expert nurse specialist.

When you first discover you have advanced metastatic breast cancer there can sometimes be a wave of hopelessness and a feeling that there is no point in thinking about any more treatment. But this would be a great mistake. Although the situation is incurable it is usually very far from being terminal. These days many women with advanced breast cancer live for years and years before their disease finally catches up with them, and usually for most of those years they will enjoy a good quality of life and be able to live a full and active existence very close to, if not the same as, they were used to before. This means that having treatment with hormones or cytotoxic drugs can make a great difference both in terms of how you feel, easing symptoms like pain and sickness, and also offering the possibility of years of extra life. So it is well worth exploring with your oncologist what your choices are and what they feel is best for you.

One difference in this situation compared with when you are having treatment for a primary breast cancer is that your oncologist knows the condition cannot be cured and will make a great effort not only to offer treatment that gives the best possible chance of increasing your life expectancy but also to ensure that the treatment they give leads to a good quality of life for you. So keeping side effects to a minimum and offering other drugs and treatments that relieve any symptoms will be very important in ensuring that you feel as fit as possible and get the most out of life even though you are still having treatment.

Conclusion

Forty years ago I was in a taxi going to the Christie Hospital in Manchester and the driver asked me if I thought there would ever be a cure for cancer. I explained that many cancers could already be cured and that in breast cancer half of all women who had the disease survived. Last year a taxi driver in Wolverhampton asked me the same question and this time I was able to tell him that more than 8 out of 10 women with breast cancer are cured. This dramatic improvement in outcome is good news, and even for those women who are unlucky enough for their cancer to come back the reality is that many will be able to live a relatively normal life for a number of years as a result of modern-day treatment.

Improvement in treatment, in particular the development of new drugs and new ways of using those drugs, is what has led to the increased chance of cure for women with early breast cancer and the increased life expectancy for those with advanced disease. In fact you could say that these days oncologists are spoilt for choice when it comes to deciding the best treatment to recommend for someone with breast cancer. On the one hand this is a very good situation to be in but on the other it does create a problem – choices have to be made and that isn't always easy.

A few months ago one of my fellow oncologists, who specializes in lung cancer, told me that he had sat in on a meeting of breast cancer experts and had been quite amazed that they spent the entire time arguing about what were the best treatments. I was not surprised. The uncertainty, the debates, the arguments among breast oncologists are not because nothing can be done but because there are so many different treatment options, all of which give very similar, very good, results. But at the end of the day decisions do have to be made: your oncologist cannot sit in a clinic and say, 'Here we are Ms Jones, there are five different treatments that are just as good as each other' and stop there. They have to decide which one of those five treatments they are actually going to use.

Doctors are human (I know that may be hard to believe but I promise you it is true). This means they are not all the same and different oncologists will handle this situation differently. Some will have very clear-cut views on what they think is right and confidently give you definite advice; they may not even tell you that you have a choice, although they should. Others will spell out what the different possibilities are and suggest what they feel might be best for you, although giving you the final choice. Others will describe each of the options, discuss their advantages and disadvantages and then leave the decision entirely in your hands.

To help you make up your mind you may also have a chat with a breast specialist nurse and will almost certainly be given written information in the form of booklets or factsheets. But that written information will only tell you more about the different treatments, it won't tell you what is the right treatment for you or what you should do.

The aim of the modern-day NHS is to put the patient at the centre of decision-making; your medical team tells you what is available and what the benefits and risks are, but what happens next is up to you. Many women facing the enormous stress of a cancer diagnosis will find that looking at the evidence, weighing up the facts, balancing all the various pros and cons, and arriving at a carefully thought-through decision is just too much. They will opt for either a 'gut reaction', taking the advice of friends or family, or leave the final decision to their doctor. So long as they feel happy with this, any of these ways of handling things is fine. But the important thing is to realize that you do have a choice – the decisions about your treatment are yours to make if you want to. You have control. It is your life, your body, your cancer and you are the one who will live with the consequences of that choice.

That last phrase is important, especially when it comes to drug treatment. Saying yes to a course of chemotherapy may lead to treatment lasting some months and agreeing to hormone treatment may involve taking drugs for 5–8 years. But if you find you are struggling to cope, if you run into problems you had not expected or if there is anything about the treatment you are unhappy with, you have every right to discuss it with your doctors and reconsider. They may able to offer solutions or alternatives but if you are still unhappy then you can say no. If you think that the upset and distress of having the treatment is not worth the possible benefit then the fact that you agreed to that treatment months or years before doesn't mean that you have got to see it through come what may.

Every one of us is different – our genetic makeup, our emotional landscape, our family circumstances and our view on life all contribute to forming who we are. This means that in a crisis situation like having cancer, each of us will have different feelings and different needs. For some women, taking every possible option to get the greatest chance of a cure is all important, no matter what the side effects or inconvenience of treatment. For others, quality of life will be the most important consideration. Everyone will have their own balance between the benefits and drawbacks of therapy. When it comes to deciding about treatment, just realizing that there are choices to be made may be too much to cope with and leaving it up to your doctor may be what you feel happiest with. If that is what seems right for you then that is absolutely fine. But you may want to have more say in things, more control over what is happening to you in a situation where it is all too easy to feel that everything is out of control. And that is the point of this book: to let you know that you do have choices, you do have a voice in the decisions that are made about you and your care and your cancer, and to try and give you some of the background information to help you with making those all-important decisions.

Useful addresses

Breast Cancer Care
5–13 Great Suffolk Street
London SE1 0NS
Tel.: 0845 092 0800
Website: www.breastcancercare.org.uk

The helpline is staffed by specialist breast-care nurses; and there is printed information for anyone affected by breast cancer. The organization also provides a support service where women with breast cancer can be put in touch with a trained individual who has had personal experience of the condition.

Cancer Research UK
Angel Building
407 St John Street
London EC1V 4AD
Tel.: 020 7242 0200
Helpline: 0808 800 4040 (9 a.m. to 5 p.m., Monday to Friday)
Website: www.cancerresearchuk.org

Macmillan Cancer Support
89 Albert Embankment
London SE1 7UQ
Tel.: 020 7840 7840
Helpline: 0808 808 00 00 (9 a.m. to 8 p.m., Monday to Friday)
Website: www.macmillan.org.uk

In addition to funding cancer nursing services and offering valuable advice on coping with the financial consequences of cancer, this organization provides a number of very informative publications on breast cancer. The helpline is staffed by experienced nurses who can give further information and support.

Maggie's Centres
First Floor
One Waterloo Street
Glasgow G2 6AY
Tel.: 0300 123 1801
Website: www.maggiescentres.org

Located throughout the country, Maggie's Centres (nine at present, with more planned) are places to turn to for help with any of problems related to cancer. Under one roof you can get information, advice about benefits, and emotional support. You don't have to make an appointment, and everything is free of charge. There is also a specific online centre for those who are not able to access one of the other centres. The website contains extensive information on how the centres can help. The job of the professionals at Maggie's is to listen to you – to help you find out what you want and give you what you need to help yourself.

Index